NMS *Review for the Clinical Skills Assessment Exam*

NMS *Review for the Clinical Skills Assessment Exam*

Erich A. Arias, MD

University of Monterrey
Health Sciences Division—School of Medicine
Monterrey, Mexico

PGY-1, Surgery
Department of Surgery
University of Nevada—School of Medicine
Las Vegas, Nevada

Editor: Elizabeth A. Nieginski
Editorial Director: Julie P. Scardiglia
Development Editor: Beth Goldner
Managing Editor: Amy Dinkel
Marketing Manager: Kelley Ray

351 West Camden Street
Baltimore, Maryland 21201-2436 USA

530 Walnut Street
Philadelphia, Pennsylvania 19106 USA

Printed in the United States of America

ISBN: 0-7817-2542-9

We'd like to hear from you! If you have comments or suggestions regarding this Lippincott Williams & Wilkins title, please contact us at the appropriate customer service number listed below, or send correspondence to **book_comments@lww.com.** If possible, please remember to include your mailing address, phone number, and a reference to the book title and author in your message. To purchase additional copies of this book call our customer service department at **(800) 638-3030** or fax orders to **(301) 824-7390.** International customers should call **(301) 714-2324.**

3 4 5 6 7 8 9 10

Reviewers

—————•

Chapter 3

Ophthalmology
Henry Miller, MD
Autonomous University of Chihuahua, Chihuahua, Mexico
Ophthalmology, Asociacion Para Evitar la Ceguera en Mexico, IAP
National Autonomous University of Mexico, Mexico DF, Mexico
Hospital Clínica del Parque, Chihuahua, Mexico

Internal Medicine
Arturo Castro, MD
Mayor National University of Saint Marcos, Lima, Peru
Internal Medicine, University of Tennessee, Memphis, TN
Family Health Medical Center, Wautoma, Wisconsin

Surgery
Gonzalo Jimenez, MD
University of Monterrey, Monterrey, Mexico
Department of Surgery, Hospital 25, Instituto Mexicano de Seguridad Social
Autonomous University of New Lion, Monterrey, Mexico

Family Practice
Jesus Blanco, MD
University of Monterrey, Monterrey, Mexico
Hospital Clínica del Parque, Chihuahua, Mexico

Orthopedics
Edmundo Berumen, MD
Autonomous University of Chihuahua, Chihuahua, Mexico
Orthopedic Surgery, MacMaster University, Hamilton, Ontario, Canada
Hospital Clínica del Parque, Chihuahua, Mexico

Chapter 4

Obstetrics and Gynecology
Jesus Leal del Rosal, MD
Military School of Medicine, Mexico
Obstetrics and Gynecology, Miami Valley Hospital, Dayton, Ohio
Chairman of the American College of Obstetricians and Gynecologists, District VII,
    Mexico
Professor of Medicine, Autonomous University of Chihuahua
Hospital Clínica del Parque, Chihuahua, Mexico

Carlos Leal, MD
University of Monterrey, Monterrey, Mexico
Obstetrics and Gynecology, Hospital Clínica del Parque-Aunonomous University of
    Chihuahua, Chihuahua, Mexico
Fellow in Gynecology Oncology, University of Otawa, Otawa, Canada

Fernando Noriega Ruckauf, MD
Saint Martin of Porras University, Lima, Peru
Obstetrics and Gynecology, Hospital Guillermo Almenara, Lima, Peru
Fellowship in Infertility and Assisted Reproduction, CEGYR-University of Buenos Aires, Argentina

Chapter 5

Neurology
Barney J. Stern, MD
Professor, Department of Neurology
Emory University School of Medicine
Atlanta, Georgia

Chapter 6

Psychiatry
Silvia Drumond, MD
University of Monterrey, Monterrey, Mexico
Psychiatry, University of Texas at Galveston, Galveston, Texas

Chapter 7

Pediatrics
Manuel Gutierrez, MD
Peruvian University Cayetano Heredia, Lima, Peru
Auxiliary Professor of Pediatrics, Peruvian University Cayetano Heredia
Pediatrics, SUNY Health Science Center at Brooklyn, Brooklyn, New York
Fellowship in Pediatric Pulmonology

Chapter 9

Immigration Issues
Silvia Arias, Attorney at Law
Peruvian Catholic University, Peru
Masters in Law, University of Texas, Austin, Texas
e-mail: sarias00@yahoo.com

John Paul Barber, Attorney at Law
University of Mississippi, Jackson, Mississippi
e-mail: jpbarber@intop.net

General Review

Norma A. Perez, MD
University of Monterrey, Monterrey, Mexico
Rehabilitation Medicine, National University Autonomous of Mexico, Mexico
Research Associate, Center for Society and Population Health School of Public Health, University of Texas Health Science Center, Houston, Texas

Sandra Olivier
Business Management
Miami, Florida

Index

Dedication

———•

To my mother and father, Rosa and Eduardo, whose unceasing love and support pointed me in the right direction for my life and professional endeavors.

To my brothers, Silvia and Eduardo, for all the time shared together as a family.

To my wife, Fiorella, whose lifelong love, support, and patience has made everything possible.

To all international medical graduates who are pursuing entry into a residency program in the United States.

Contents

-------•

Preface

For an international medical graduate (IMG) who aspires to obtain graduate medical education (GME) in the United States, the obstacles seem tremendous. Not only do you have to pass the USMLE boards and the TOEFL test with high scores, but you also have to demonstrate your clinical skills in a simulated scenario—the Clinical Skills Assessment exam, or the CSA.

Many IMGs successfully obtained internships and medical residencies in American hospitals years before. However, from the viewpoint of GME programs and the Educational Commission for Foreign Medical Graduates (ECFMG®), an apparent disparity between IMGs and United States medical graduates was evident. The complaints were not focused on lack of clinical knowledge; instead, they focused on the foreign medical graduate's ability to communicate with the patient appropriately and compose a pertinent patient medical note (patient note).

On July 1, 1998, the ECFMG® introduced the Clinical Skills Assessment (CSA) exam, a new and final evaluation for ECFMG® certification. At this time, the CSA exam does not have a final quantitative score. Instead, this exam is being evaluated based on a structural checklist filled out by the standardized patients (SPs) . The SP does not subjectively rate the IMGs clinical skills; to be more precise, the SP objectively documents whether or not the IMG asked the appropriate questions and performed the proper physical exam maneuvers on the checklist. Patient note-taking skills are rated based on organization of information, data interpretation, tentative diagnoses (differential diagnosis), and the ordering of pertinent diagnostic tests. Interpersonal skills and spoken English proficiency are also evaluated and added together to the IMG's final score. For this reason, this exam has only *Pass* or *Fail* score results.

This book is not intended to be a comprehensive textbook. It is intended to be a guide and clinical review preparation for the CSA exam. There are other books on the market that are useful to review the clinical assessment, but no one book has the direct and concise focus on the CSA exam.

This book contains everything the ECFMG® recognizes that IMGs frequently lack in comparison to United States medical graduates. For this reason, this book is the perfect choice if you want to pass the CSA exam. Many IMGs come from English-speaking countries and many do not. Regardless, it is important for an IMG to know how American physicians compose medical notes. For example, instead of saying or writing *complete blood count* and *myocardial infarction,* an American physician will say and write *CBC* and *MI,* respectively. Writing a patient note will vary depending on the disciplines you face during the CSA exam; saving time and how you write your patient notes are crucial factors to succeeding on the exam.

In summary, this book is the only one that can teach you how to transmit the medical information as needed in real clinical practice as the CSA demands and as future interns or residents will need. The goals of this book are 1) to review important aspects of the clinical exam and medical history in different disciplines and then 2) to teach you how to compose a written medical note the way United States health care providers do in clinical practice.

This book contains many figures and tables to highlight important concepts in different disciplines. After two brief introductory chapters, Chapter 3 covers important aspects about internal medicine, family practice, surgery, and orthopedics. Also, there is an entire chapter about the application process for residency programs in United States hospitals as well as coverage of various immigration issues.

I encourage readers to suggest improvements and identify deficiencies, and I hope that this book will be useful for achieving your goals and for completing your medical education in the United States.

Erich A. Arias, MD

Acknowledgments

—————•

I would like to express my deepest appreciation to Elizabeth Nieginski, Amy Dinkel, and Beth Goldner of Lippincott Williams & Wilkins for making this project happen and for all of their editorial attention.

I would also like to express my special thanks to Dr. Norma Perez who gave liberally of her time and knowledge. I also express gratitude to the many physicians involved in the review process of this book for their invaluable feedback. And lastly, I would like to thank my parents, brothers, and wife for their priceless support and confidence.

1

Basic Tools for the Clinical Skills Assessment Exam

INTRODUCTION

Performing a correct clinical examination is directly associated with learning how to write a correct medical record. The general rule is to start with the patient interview and then continue with the physical exam. Frequently, a great amount of data is obtained during the interview process, and the rest of the information is added during the physical exam.

In medical school, you should have learned the steps necessary to take a complete medical history. In the United States, it is very important to record everything in the medical record. The legal issues that medical professionals may face demand that physicians are accurate during clinical exams and cautious about what is written in the medical record. Furthermore, U.S. medical schools try to have similar training programs and evaluations regarding how to create a well-organized and well-documented medical record. Some foreign medical schools are very competitive, and their students spend a balanced time in learning theory and in clinical practice; on the other hand, other foreign medical schools may spend more time in clinical practice than in theory and vice versa. The disparity between these training regimens became apparent when the Educational Commission of Foreign Medical Graduates (ECFMG®) combined all international medical graduates (IMGs) into one group. After a decade of analyzing the differences, the ECFMG® changed the requirements for the certification of all IMGs. In 1998, the Clinical Skills Assessment (CSA) exam was established as a prerequisite for ECFMG® certification. Many factors influence a student's score: the student's written and spoken English skills, the physician-patient relationship demonstrated during the CSA exam, and the student's familiarity with American medical terminology. For CSA exam purposes, you will need to be acquainted with questions and analysis, as physicians are with real patients.

The Basics of the CSA Exam

It is very important to organize your time. You will have 25 minutes to interact with the standardized patient (SP) and to write a medical note. A maximum of 15 minutes is permitted to interact with the SP in the examination room; the remaining 10 minutes are used to compose the medical note. **If you complete your SP examination in less than 15 minutes, you will have additional time to write your note.** You will have

1

encounters with 11 patients; 10 of these encounters will be scored. The nonscoreable encounter will be used for research purposes. The materials that you must bring with you on the day of the CSA exam are your stethoscope and lab coat.

Before you enter each examination room, you will have a few minutes to review some information about the SP; the SP's name, gender, vital signs, and reason for the visit will be posted on the examination room door. This is known as the **doorway information sheet.** After you have reviewed the doorway information, an announcement will let you know when you can start the test. All SPs will be adults. In some cases, however, they will be discussing problems related to their children. SPs vary in terms of age, gender, and ethnicity. The regimens presented during the CSA exam are illustrated in this book and are presented in Table 1–1.

One advantage is that you will not encounter a truly ill patient, even if the SP simultaneously presents with real abnormal findings. For example, the SP may present with real residual hemiplegia as a result of a stroke, but the reason for the consultation can be a sore throat and therefore you are to focus on his sore throat complaint. Another advantage is that you will not have to deal with pediatric patients.

The disadvantage is that you will deal with actors who are specifically trained to challenge you. The SPs are not medical personnel; they are prepared to represent a specific clinical condition and simulate clinical signs and symptoms concerning that complaint. Some patients/SPs may be presented to you with acute, subacute, and chronic problems.

Perform the physical exam as you would with a real patient, with one exception— you will not perform a pelvic, rectal, genital, or female breast examination. Everything in the CSA exam is intended to challenge you as in real clinical practice. Time is a key feature, and organization will be your key to success.

During the interview and physical exam, you will gather information from the SP necessary to form a tentative diagnosis. Start a relationship with the SP as you do with a real patient. Try to help him or her to trust and confide in you. During the interview and physical exam forget that you are being evaluated. However, always be careful with the time you have and with every step you take during the questioning and examination. You must be prepared to make a well-organized and concise medical note. Make the appropriate notes according to the cases presented. Organize yourself well enough to compose a complete medical note and also be familiar with some standard writing formats from different disciplines according to your patient's needs. The elements that you will need to obtain and include in the medical history will depend on the cases presented. Table 1–2 shows some important aspects that should always be kept in mind.

Not every section of the medical history needs to be included in your notes; use your own criteria case by case. If you believe that the SP needs to be examined on one particular area (e.g., chest examination), focus your exam on this area without forgetting to ask about and examine other body parts or systems in a general manner.

An announcement will inform you when there are only 5 minutes left before finishing time. Try to close the interview before the time indicated.

The diagnostic workup should be oriented to formulating a tentative diagnosis. The information gathered during the medical history and physical exam will provide you with a framework and clues for understanding the patient's problem. Figure 1–1 shows how to organize all this information.

TABLE 1–1. Regimens Presented During the CSA Exam

General	Obstetrics and Gynecology	Nervous System	Pediatrics
Internal medicine, family practice, surgery, and orthopedics	Obstetrics and gynecology	Neurology, psychiatry	Pediatrics

TABLE 1–2. Elements to Remember during an Encounter with a Standardized Patient

The Interview	The Physical Exam	The Written Note
Always introduce yourself	Always wash your hands before examining the patient†	Be precise and concise
Always remember the patient's name	Always explain to the patient the maneuvers you are going to perform	Record the events in the order in which they occurred
Make appropriate eye contact, preferably at the patient's eye level	Never examine the patient through the gown	Use only well-known abbreviations
Start with facilitation* or open-ended questions*	Use the extension table when needed	Write important positives and negatives related to the medical history information and physical findings (positive tests)
Do not confront,* rush, or cut off patient's dialogue	Perform a focused physical exam	
Always answer the patient's questions	Do not perform genital, rectal, or breast examinations	
Explain to the SP your tentative impression and plan for diagnosis		
Do not use medical terminology to explain something to the SP		
When pertinent, counsel the SP about preventive measures and risk factor reduction		

* See the section on Interviewing Techniques in this chapter.
† For the purposes of this book, SP and patient are used interchangeably.

ENGLISH COMMUNICATION SKILLS

If you grew up in an English-speaking country, you can skip this section. Communicating in English is difficult. Learning to communicate in English is a long process that not only depends on passing a single test or tests, but also on other factors that influence your understanding of common, spoken English. The ECFMG® (in conjunction with the introduction of the CSA exam) implemented the Test of English as a Foreign Language (TOEFL) in 1999 as a single method to evaluate IMGs. Before that, TOEFL was an alternative to the ECFMG® English test. The computer-based TOEFL test replaces

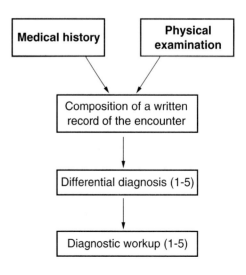

FIGURE 1–1. Organization of information from the medical history and physical examination, leading to the diagnostic workup.

the ECFMG® English test. The TOEFL test also evaluates writing skills. A minimum score of 213 is necessary to fulfill the ECFMG® requirements.

Apart from any study method or evaluation for understanding common American English, it is necessary to have a "good ear." This ability can only be obtained by a great deal of practicing, listening, and speaking. During the CSA exam, your spoken English skills will be evaluated by all SPs that you encounter. Pronunciation and the amount of effort required by the SPs to understand you will be considered and incorporated in your score. If you have any doubt about your proficiency in English, the ECFMG® recommends that you take the Test of Spoken English (TSE). This test was developed by the Educational Testing Service (ETS) and is useful as a screening test only. Studies indicate that if your score on the TSE is lower than 35, it is more likely that you will not be able to demonstrate the appropriate spoken English necessary to pass the CSA exam. (However, a score above 35 does not ensure that you will pass the CSA exam.) The following recommendations may help you to increase your English vocabulary and to "tune" your ear.

If you are living in an English-speaking country:

1. Try to speak with native English speakers as often as possible.
2. If you already speak relatively fluent English, work on your pronunciation and accent.
3. Whenever possible, try to think in English. It is a good sign if you start the day dreaming or thinking in English.
4. Watch or listen to news reports, weather reports, and documentary programs on television or radio.
5. Attend live lectures at your school, college, or university. If accessible, use the language laboratory at your school.
6. Make and answer telephone calls. Request any information that you need using the telephone. Do not ask someone else to assist you. Use all opportunities to practice speaking English.

If you are living in a non–English-speaking country:

1. Take a formal English course at your local institute, college, or university. Start to study English months or years before you plan to take the CSA exam. If possible, take the course during your medical school years or before.
2. Whenever possible, try to speak with native English speakers. Go to the tourist attractions in your area and try to meet English-speaking foreigners. By doing this, you will improve your English skills and act as a good host of your own country.
3. If you have access to cable or satellite television, try to watch American channels. Listen to how they talk, the tones, the idioms, etc. Start with commercials, weather reports, and documentaries.
4. If you have a television with closed captioning, use it to see how certain words are spelled. Captioning also helps you to increase your vocabulary.
5. Avoid watching American movies with written translations to your language (i.e., subtitles). Closed captioning is better than a translation.

INTERVIEWING TECHNIQUES

There are several ways to assess the patient/SP. Everyone has their own way to approach a patient, but it is important to know the essential parts of an interview. It is also necessary to know how the patient's expectations are influenced by his or her cultural background, previous experiences, personality, and present physical and mental status.

Facilitation. "*How can I help you?*" "*And then what happened?*" Questions such as these provide the patient with an opportunity to explain the main problem or complaint in his or her own words.

Open-ended questions. "*Tell me about your pain.*" This type of question provides some orientation to the patient, encouraging him or her to speak freely but directed to the main problem. Here you can obtain a great amount of oriented information. This type of questioning is often followed by facilitation and also produces a good physician-patient relationship.

Direct questioning. *"On what side of your chest do you feel the pain?"* You can use this type of questioning if you want to focus on the chief complaint. These types of questions will save you a great deal of time. You can use this type of question during the CSA examination, which will also facilitate your review.

Empathy. *"I understand that you are worried about the consequences of your injury."* Let the patient know that you understand his or her problem as if it had occurred to you.

Support. *"It must have been a terrible experience for you."* Let the patient know that you comprehend his or her feelings.

Confrontation. *"Do you really believe that the explanation that you told me is the cause of your problems?"* Never use this kind of question on the CSA examination. This type of question draws the patient's attention to his or her inconsistencies.

Silence. Providing no response produces the worst physician-patient relationship. If for any reason an SP asks you a question and you do not know the answer, say *"I don't know."*

Validation. *"It is common that people feel exactly the way you are feeling at this moment."* Give credence to the patient's feelings.

Recapitulation. *"Let's see, you started having chest pain while you were eating last night?"* This technique is normally used at the end of the interview. This is a way of organizing all the information obtained.

Always remember that you will need to organize your ideas and questions. **Try not to think that you are being evaluated.** Your nervousness can be harmful during the process. Stay calm and organize your thoughts and your time. As in any physician-patient relationship, it is important to portray that you are sincere, human, and experienced. Above all, the physician should do all he or she can to ensure patient compliance (i.e., that the patient follows the physician's instructions regarding medications and life style changes). Table 1–3 lists factors affecting compliance. Try to achieve a posi-

TABLE 1–3. Factors Affecting Compliance

Good Compliance	Poor Compliance	Approximate % of Patients Who Are Compliant with Treatment
Good doctor-patient relationship	An indifferent perception of the doctor	33.3% not compliant with the treatment
Doctor is knowledgeable about and sensitive to the patient's beliefs	Doctor fails to explain the diagnosis or cause of the symptoms	33.3% compliant with some of the treatment
Doctor is enthusiastic	Complicated treatments	33.3% compliant with treatment
Doctor has a good amount of expertise	Change in patient's behavior in smoking, exercise schedules, etc.	
Doctor's older age*		
Short waiting room time	Long waiting room time	
Seriously ill patients	Patients who are not seriously ill	
Patients with acute illnesses who understand how medication(s) work(s)	Patients with chronic illnesses who do not understand how medication(s) work(s)	
A well written explanation on how to take medications	Verbal instructions on how to take medications	

*A patient's impression of a young physician can be that he or she is too inexperienced; thus, the role of the physician in society usually overrides that initial impression.

(Adapted with permission from Fadem B: *BRS Behavioral Science,* 2e. Philadelphia: Lippincott Williams & Wilkins, 1994, p 167–168.)

tive transference reaction (i.e., how the patient sees the doctor and his or her level of ability; in a positive reaction, the patient sees the physician with a high level of confidence and respects his or her abilities). If you have success in achieving these goals, you can improve your score.

OVERALL ASSESSMENT RECOMMENDATIONS

Be prepared to explain your findings to the patient. Never close the session with a single diagnosis. Explain to the patient what you believe he or she has, but always consider that there may be other possibilities. **Do not give false reassurance** about the prognosis. Be prepared to answer questions such as, *"Am I going to die?"* If a patient asks you a question about the prognosis at the beginning of the encounter, let the patient know that you will be able to answer any questions after having completed the clinical exam. There are many recommendations that you need to keep in mind as you examine an SP. Before a patient/SP session, prepare yourself and try to meet the following objectives:

1. Read the doorway information carefully. Focus on the chief complaint (CC), patient age, and important or abnormal values recorded with the vital signs. It is very important to remember the patient's first and last names. Then, knock on the door before you enter the examination room.
2. As you enter the examination room, introduce yourself. Call the patient by his or her name. *"Hello Mr. O'Brien. I am Dr. Bhargava. What can I do for you today?"*
3. Allow the patient to explain freely his or her reason for the office visit (facilitation). After the patient finishes, ask a direct or open-ended question, as may be necessary.
4. Always look into the patient's eyes when you speak to him or her.
5. Make the appropriate notes on the blank sheet provided to you as you proceed with the questioning.
6. Always wash your hands or use disposable gloves before examining the patient. Washing your hands and wearing gloves may be appropriate for a patient with a suspected immunosuppressive problem.
7. Perform a focused clinical exam. Always explain to the patient what you are going to do before you do it.
8. Be polite and courteous during any maneuvering. Do not repeat painful maneuvers.
9. As you finish the examination, help the SP to put his or her gown back on.
10. Explain your findings and your tentative diagnosis to the patient. Do not use medical terminology. Depending on the patient's background, it may be easy for him or her to understand some medical terms. For some patients, it may be more appropriate to use more simple words. Use your own judgment. *"Ms. Carter, I believe that you may have a urinary tract infection but it also could be a kidney stone."*
11. Explain to the patient if further study or laboratory tests are necessary. Remember that for CSA purposes, a pelvic-rectal examination must be considered a diagnostic workup plan. Explaining tests and their importance is always helpful.
12. Before leaving the room, ask the patient/SP if he or she has any questions. Common questions about prognosis include, *"Do I have cancer?" "Am I going to die?" "This chest pain is an infarction?"*
13. Terminate the session properly. Leave the examining room and then proceed to composing the written note.

2

The Real Medical Note

INTRODUCTION

The medical record is a legal document that contains medical notes that record medical data; record results of discussions with the patient and family; and document and record consents, living wills, advance directives, and resuscitation wishes. It is very important to know what you can and cannot write in the medical note. Remember, everything you write on a medical note is subject to review if the law requires it.

It is important to know how to write a medical note, not only because it is part of the daily medical practice but also because it is part of the medical education and curriculum for most United States medical students. Writing a medical note has recently been included as part of the new examination—the Clinical Skills Assessment (CSA)—for international medical graduates (IMGs). The medical notes that you learned to compose during your medical school training differ greatly from the medical notes that you will need to write as an intern or resident in the United States. For example, in some countries a small note is considered sufficient. In other countries, such as the United States, complete documentation is mandatory. During your first encounter in a United States hospital, you will see the differences from the real medical note and the samples you have seen in textbooks.

WRITING MEDICAL NOTES

The main purpose of the medical note is to transmit any specific information to other health care providers, including other physicians, nurses, pharmacists, nutritionists, and physician's assistants. Recording information can often be problematic because, in part, physicians frequently forget how to write in a correct form (i.e., well-organized, clear, and easily understandable English). The function of the medical note is to record the **history, physical examination,** and **laboratory findings.** It also serves to discuss findings and document new events, procedures, operations, treatments, and plans. The following section contains a list of recommendations for writing medical notes.

GENERAL RECOMMENDATIONS FOR WRITING MEDICAL NOTES

The following recommendations are general tips to consider when you are writing a medical note.

Style Issues

1. Use clear, understandable writing and words.
2. Complete the necessary data that identifies you as an examiner.
3. Record the information in a logical sequence.
4. Include pertinent positive and negative features.

Measurements of Value, Terminology, and Abbreviations

1. Record the vital signs as **temperature (T°), blood pressure (BP), heart rate (HR),** and **respiratory rate (RR).** You can also record HR as pulse (P) and RR as respirations (R). Normally the vital signs are on the **doorway information sheet** posted on the examination room door. You are expected to accept this information as correct. But you can recheck the vital signs if you feel it is necessary.
2. Become familiar with degrees Fahrenheit. This temperature measurement of value is the standard in the United States. As stated by the ECFMG®, temperature information will be recorded in both Celsius and Fahrenheit on the doorway information sheet. Knowing temperature equivalencies is helpful, because a standardized patient (SP) may communicate temperature changes that have occurred. Table 2–1 lists some important equivalencies.
3. Become familiar with weights in pounds (1 kg = 2.2 lb). For practical purposes, divide the weight in pounds by 2. This will provide a rough estimate of the weight in kilograms.
4. Use precise medical terminology in your comments. Be succinct and specific to the problem. For example, it is better to write *dyspnea* than *shortness of breath, leg* than *lower extremity, subepigastric pain* than *abdominal or stomach pain,* or *hesitancy* than *delay in the initiation of micturition.*
5. Use abbreviations commonly used in the United States (see Appendix). The abbreviations most commonly used in the United States are defined throughout this book. Study them so that you will be familiar with them.

   Using abbreviations is a common practice in U.S. health care institutions. For example, instead of saying or writing, "Complete blood count, methicillin-resistant *Staphylococcus aureus,* chronic heart failure, or shortness of breath," it is common to say or write, "CBC, MERSA, CHF and SOB," respectively.
6. Learn the following standard abbreviations most commonly used in written medical notes and medical prescriptions:

   bid = two times per day
   tid = three times per day
   qid = four times per day
   QD = once a day
   PO = by mouth, orally
   IV = intravenous
   IM = intramuscular
   SC = subcutaneous
   u/d = single dose
   PRN = taken or administered as needed

TABLE 2–1. Important Temperature Equivalencies

Normal	98.6°F = 37°C
Fever	100.4°F = 38°C
	102.2°F = 39°C
	104°F = 40°C

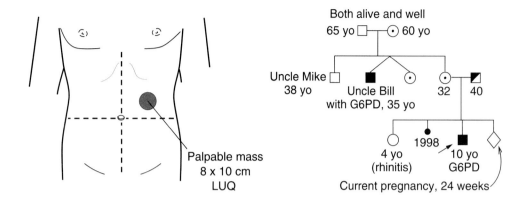

A. Abdominal diagram   **B. Family pedigree diagram**

FIGURE 2–1. Diagrams used to explain findings in a schematic form. **A)** Schematic representation of the finding of an abdominal mass during a physical examination. **B)** Family pedigree diagram. Refer to Figure 3–2 in Chapter 3 for detailed information about pedigree symbols. G6PD = glucose-6-phosphate dehydrogenase deficiency; yo = years old.

7. Know how to summarize the results of common laboratory tests by using the common stick figures used in United States (see Figure 3–16 in Chapter 3). If you consider it pertinent, use diagrams to be explicit; this will also save time. For example, you can draw diagrams to explain a particular finding on the correspondent anatomic area or to address other important data (Figure 2–1).

Important Information to Include

1. Include pertinent positive and negative findings. And try to quantify symptoms and clinical findings commonly used in the United States (Table 2–2).
2. Consider the importance of weighing the SP according to his or her clinical condition. For example, if you suspect that the SP has chronic heart failure (CHF) or you encounter a pregnant SP, you should weigh the SP and document the findings.
3. Apply clinical tests that you consider related to the problem. Remember that part of the evaluation is based on how you perform the tests.
4. Perform a quick neurologic exam if you consider it necessary. But remember, you cannot do this for all SPs—only those with positive neurologic symptoms.
5. Add to your medical note, if necessary, such things as, "*CBC pending, ultrasound pending, urinalysis pending.*" This indicates that you have not yet received the results of the corresponding tests.

TABLE 2–2. Measurement of Clinical Findings

Symptom/Finding	Quantifying Terms or Symbols
Pain	Mild, moderate, severe
Reflexes	0 to 4 (4+ = hyperactive, 0= no response)
Edema	1 to 4 (1 = slight, 4 = severe)
Pulses	1 to 4 (1 = decreased but palpable, 4 = pounding)
Murmurs	1 to 6 (1 = hard to hear, 6 = heard without stethoscope)
Chest pain	1 to 10 (1 = slight, 10 = described as "worst in my life" by the patient)

6. Record *how* the patient has been taking medication if applicable. For example, tracking antibiotic treatment can be recorded as follows: *dicloxacillin 500 mg day 5/10, PO qid.* This means that the SP is on the fifth day of 10 prescribed days of dicloxacillin treatment, taken by the oral route three times per day.
7. Track major events in the care of the SP—e.g., postsurgery day 2 or MICU (medical intensive care unit) day 3.

Pitfalls to Avoid

1. Avoid criticizing other colleagues' opinions or diagnoses within the medical note.
2. Do include bibliographic references.
3. Do not highlight personal opinions about the patient, such as criticizing the patient's behavior.

3.

Writing Medical Notes and the Physical Examination

INTRODUCTION

Before you start reading this chapter, it is very important that you relax. The clinical skills assessment (CSA) examination is designed to represent common cases that you may see in general practice. The CSA exam is not as stressful as the USMLE boards.

On the CSA exam, "how you do" and "what you do" are very important. You never will have time to perform a complete medical history. Perform your clinical exam and write notes that are oriented to the problem, without forgetting important findings that the patient might reveal upon questioning. Performing complicated tests or saturating the patient with questions are not recommended.

When you compose a medical note, it will vary according to the clinical situation that the standardized patient (SP) is going to simulate. An SP who presents to you having an acute problem will not be the same as an SP who is presenting with a chronic disease. Furthermore, you might encounter patients with actual abnormal findings that are not necessarily their principal reason of visit.

You need to write your patient notes according to the particular case. Not every part of the medical history needs to be taken in every case. This chapter gives you the opportunity to learn about the general format for medical notes that the ECFMG® recommends using on the CSA exam.

This chapter serves as a matrix model for all medical history formats discussed through this book. Some specialties have their own particular characteristics, which are covered in separate chapters; however, in reality, they would all be included here. As in real practice, you need to accommodate your questioning, physical examination, and patient notes on a case-by-case basis. The CSA test is designed to be administered in a limited time period; if you are not organized in your approach, you might lose time and then points to your favor.

Figure 3–1 is the general format of the parameters of a medical note for the CSA exam. As stated by the ECFMG®, not all the parameters are necessarily pertinent to every case. Your own criterion is very important and is part of your evaluation and score. Write a medical note according to the data obtained from the patient and the physical examination you perform. Address important positive and negative findings, questions (e.g., about risk factors), and maneuvering results.

Every section of this patient note format might be developed, reviewing important aspects of the physical exam, questioning and writing notes. For the purposes of this chapter, every example of a medical note is classified:

```
┌─────────────────────────────────────────────────────────────────┐
│                                                                   │
│  A) MEDICAL HISTORY              B) PHYSICAL EXAMINATION           │
│     1. Chief complaint (CC)         1. General examination (GE)    │
│     2. History of the present       2. HEENT                       │
│        illness (HPI)                3. Neck                        │
│     3. Past medical history (PMH)   4. Chest ---► Respiratory system│
│     4. Social history (SH)                  ---► Heart            │
│     5. Family history (FH)          5. Abdomen                     │
│     6. Review of systems (ROS)      6. Male genitalia             │
│                                     7. Neurologic                 │
│                                     8. Musculoskeletal            │
│                                     9. Other                       │
│                                                                   │
│  C) DIFFERENTIAL DIAGNOSIS        D) DIAGNOSTIC WORKUP             │
│     –Plans for dif. diagnosis (1-5)  –Plans for diagnosis (1-5)    │
│                                      –Plans for rectal/pelvic/female│
│                                       breast                       │
│                                                                   │
└─────────────────────────────────────────────────────────────────┘
```

FIGURE 3–1. General format of a patient note. The chief complaint will be provided on the doorway information sheet as an opening scenario. **Remember, in the CSA exam you are not allowed to perform a genital examination.** HEENT = head, eyes, ears, nose, throat.

Gen (general) includes surgery, internal medicine, and so forth
Ob/Gyn (obstetrics and gynecology)
P (pediatrics)

The medical note classification (Gen, Ob/Gyn, P) is only used as a reference of what had been written on it. It is not intended to be specific for any of those disciplines (internal medicine, surgery, pediatrics, obstetrics and gynecology, etc.). Furthermore, there are individual chapters for obstetrics and gynecology, pediatrics, neurology, and psychiatry.

MEDICAL HISTORY

Every part of the medical history in Figure 3–1 is covered in this chapter. Relevant physical findings and their correlation with clinical pathology are discussed. Tables and figures are provided to assist you. The written note examples are important tools that will help you compose your own written notes when you need to do it and as the CSA demands. Abbreviations will be used gradually. If you do not know the meaning of any abbreviation, see the Appendix.

Chief Complaint

The chief complaint (CC) helps you orient to the principal information about the patient. Questions such as, *What is the purpose of your visit?,* are very informative. During the CSA exam, you receive information about the patient, including his name, age, ethnicity, gender, presence of major illnesses, and the immediate problem—i.e., the chief complaint. This information is posted on the **doorway information sheet** before you enter the room to see the SP. This information is important and may provide clues to the final diagnoses. See the following examples:

Chief Complaint (Gen)

Mr. Barnett is a 26-year-old male with insulin-dependent diabetes mellitus (IDDM) who is admitted because of altered mental status.

Chief Complaint (Gen)

Mr. Garza is a 58-year-old (yo) Hispanic male, who is currently in treatment for hypertension (HTN), chronic heart failure (CHF), and non-insulin-dependent diabetes mellitus (NIDDM), who came complaining of shortness of breath.

C. Complaint (Ob/Gyn)

Ms. Garland is a 19 yo black (b) female, previously well, who came to the emergency room with abdominal pain, chills and vaginal bleeding.

CC (P)

This is a 3 yo boy who came showing irritability and abdominal discomfort. Mother states that he has a fever of 38°C, diarrhea, and abdominal pain.

History of the Present Illness (HPI)

The HPI is the history of the present illness, not the history of all of the patient's illnesses. The HPI should be a clear, accurate, and specific description of the present problem and its relation with any other events or medical problems. In a narrative and chronological form, the HPI should include the onset of the problem, the scenario in which it was developed, its manifestations, treatments, and its impact on the patient's life. The principal symptoms should be described in terms of:

Timing: Onset, duration, and frequency
When did the pain start?
How long ago did the pain start?
Is the pain constant? Does it come and go?
Location
Can you point to where the pain is?
Does the pain go anywhere?
Quality: Some pains can be described as sharp, penetrating, dull, colicky, vague, etc.
How would you describe the pain?
Quantity: For most pain, you can measure the patient's complaint as mild, moderate, or severe. For chest pain, you can grade from 1–10 point scale.
Setting
Does the pain have a relation to any particular event?
Factors that aggravated or relieve the symptoms
Does your pain increase on deep inspiration?

The HPI is one of the most important parts of the medical history, but there is no predetermined format. During the CSA exam, time is scarce, so do not spend too much time addressing one particular point; be descriptive, but be precise.

See the following medical notes, so you can learn how to focus from a normal extended medical note to a more precise note as needed for the CSA exam:

History of the Present Illness (Gen) *(Extended format)*

This is a 56-year-old man complaining of chest pain that began 2 hours prior to presenting to the Emergency Department. The pain began during the night when he was sleeping. Nausea and diaphoresis accompanied the pain but not vomiting or shortness of breath (SOB). The pain was described as grade 8, constant, well localized on the substernal region, and radiating into the neck, upper back, and down to the left arm. He denies previous similar events, palpitations, SOB, and paroxysmal nocturnal dyspnea. He states that the pain is still there and shows no signs of remission.

HPI (Gen) *(Concise format)*

This 56 yo male (m) complains of sudden grade 8 chest pain that awoke him during the night. The pain is constant, well localized on the substernal region, radiates to the neck, upper back and L. arm. Nausea and diaphoresis were present but no vomiting, SOB, palpitations, or similar events.

History of the Present Illness (Gen) *(Extended format)*

The patient was well until one week ago when she developed nasal congestion, sore throat, and low-grade fever. These seemed to improve until 2 days ago, when she noted fever to 39°C, productive cough of green, slightly bloody colored sputum, and shortness of breath while climbing stairs. She reports diffuse muscle aches and mild nausea but denies shaking chills, chest pain, headaches, stiff neck, or abdominal pain. No recent travel, and no bird and TB exposure were reported. She reports productive chronic cough of about a teaspoon of yellowish sputum in the morning for several years but no history of lung diseases, asthma, dyspnea, or asbestos exposure.

HPI (Gen) *(Concise format)*

This patient is complaining of productive cough for several years, but 1 week ago she developed sore throat, low-grade fever, and nasal congestion. Two days ago she noted slightly bloody traces on the sputum, fever (39°C) and SOB on exercises. No TB, bird exposures, recent travel, or other important diseases were reported.

History of Present Illness (Gen) *(Extended format)*

This 64-year-old male complains of abdominal pain. The pain began vaguely this morning, initially on the midabdomen and then progressively moving until being localized on the left lower quadrant. He describes the pain as severe intermittent pain that radiates to the left groin and testicle. He also refers to having urinated this morning. He described his urine as "Coca Cola" in color. Prior to this event, he reported having sporadic similar events of pain but never like this. He self-medicated with over-the-counter analgesics. He denies previous urinary infections, cystitis, hesitancy, or frank hematuria.

HPI (Gen) *(Concise format)*

This 64 yo m is complaining of severe colic abdominal pain that initially was vaguely on the midabdomen and then moved to being well localized on the LL. quadrant. The pain radiates to the L. groin and L. testicle and he describes his morning urine as coca cola in color. He denies frank hematuria, UTIs, hesitancy, or cystitis.

History of the Present Illness (Gen) *(Extended format)*

The patient has end-stage renal disease (ESRD) due to polycystic kidney disease, treated with peritoneal dialysis for 2 years. He was otherwise well until 2 days ago when he developed confusion, decrease in the level of consciousness, palpitations, and deep respirations. The patient had been treated with diet, furosemide, and human erythropoietin. He presently refers to feeling fine and denies any alteration of his mental status. His daughter states that he recently reported having cold symptoms, and he self-medicated with his wife's Motrin. On direct questioning, his daughter confirms that the patient had reported loss of vision, tinnitus, muscle weakness, or pruritus.

HPI (Gen) *(Concise format)*

This is a patient with ESRD due to polycystic K. disease, brought by his daughter who states that he is presenting confusion, ↓ level of consciousness, palpitations, and SOB. He had been treated with dialysis, diet, furosemide, and human erythropoietin. The patient states that he feels all right, although his daughter discredits him. She states that he recently had cold symptoms and self-medicated with Motrin.

History of the Present Illness (Ob/Gyn) *(Extended Format)*

This is a 56-year-old white (w) woman complaining of urinary incontinence. The symptoms began vaguely during the course of the last three years, initially with lower abdomen heaviness sensation, and then with sporadic urinary incontinence during the night exacerbated by prolonged standing or when she lifts heavy objects. She is a postmenopausal multiparous woman, not in exogenous estrogen therapy; she denies urgency, dyspareunia, urinary tract infection (UTI), hesitancy and chronic obstructive pulmonary disease (COPD).

HPI (Ob/Gyn) *(Concise format)*

She is a 56 yo w postmenopausal woman with h/o urinary incontinence since 3 years ago. Initially the symptoms were vague and then accompanied with low abdominal heaviness sensation and standing/lifting incontinence. She denies urgency, dyspareunia, UTIs, or COPD.

Past Medical History

Document information about the patient's past medical history (PMH). This may include medical, surgical, and psychiatric history as well as screening tests. You can use the following general order for the PMH:

Past medical illnesses
Past surgical illnesses
Psychiatric illnesses
Medications
Allergies, allergies to medications
Smoking, alcohol, recreational drugs (you can include this part in social history) and HIV risk factors

See the following examples of writing the PMH in a medical note:

Past Medical History (Gen, Ob/Gyn)

10 years ago she was diagnosed with NIDDM and 5 years ago with HTN. Cholecystectomy in 1985.
Medications: Glipizide 2.5 mg QD
      Lisinopril 10 mg QD
      Aspirin prn.
Allergies: None known.

PMH (Gen)

Angina pectoris diagnosed 7 years ago, treated medically initially and then surgically with CABG in 1998 due to 3 vessel disease.
Medications: Nitroglycerin 0.6 mgs PRN
       Aspirin 325 mg QD
Allergies: Unknown

Social History

Document information about the patient's social history (SH), including occupation, marital status, social support (important in elderly), sexual orientation, religious beliefs (e.g., Jehovah Witnesses do not accept blood transfusions), and habits.

See the following examples:

Social History (Gen)

He works as a construction worker in a private company, and he is married with two children. He denies use of drugs or having extramarital affairs. Consumes alcohol (ETOH) socially, less than 3 beers/weekend. Negative HIV risk factors.

Social (Gen, Ob/Gyn)

She is divorced with two children. Works in the city of Houston as an administrator. Heterosexual, with one sexual partner. ETOH consumption occasionally, smoking positive for 1/2 pack of cigarettes/day.

SH (Gen)

He is an architect, married 1 year ago, no children. He defines himself as "straight," but referred to unprotected homosexual contacts years before.

Family History

Take the most pertinent family history (FH) information that can be related to the patient's main problem. Document the age and health (or age and cause of death) of each immediate family member, such as parents, siblings, spouse and children. Data about grandparents may be important. Document potential hereditary problems— e.g., obesity, non-insulin-dependent diabetes mellitus (NIDDM), hypertension (HTN), genetically transmitted diseases such as hemophilia and cystic fibrosis, and transmissible diseases related to a close relative such as tuberculosis. If you suspect that your patient has a genetic or familial problem, it may be necessary to make a three-generation family tree to trace the disorder. Documenting the family history in a diagram may save you time when you are writing your patient notes. Figure 3–2 shows you the symbols used to compose a pedigree. Be familiar with both forms of the following notes:

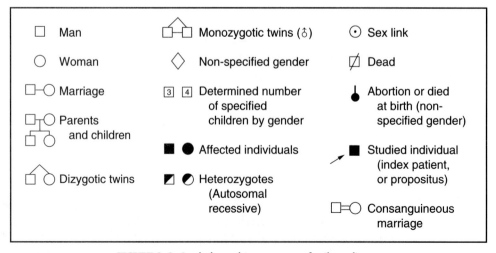

FIGURE 3–2. Symbols used to compose a family pedigree.

Family History (Gen, Ob/Gyn)

Father: Died of cerebrovascular (CVA) age 60.

Mother: Alive and well.

Brother: Alive with phobic disorder.

No cancer, DM, HTN, or heart disease.

Family Hx (Gen, Ob/Gyn)

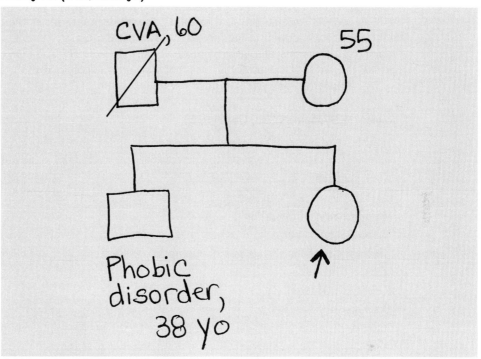

Family History (Gen, Ob/Gyn)

Father 57 yo, alive and well.

Mother 52 yo with varicose veins and migraine headaches.

The second male sibling died at birth.

Sister 29 yo, alive, ovaric tecoma resected at age of 19.

Brother 16 years old and sister 31 years old: alive and well.

Family History (Gen)

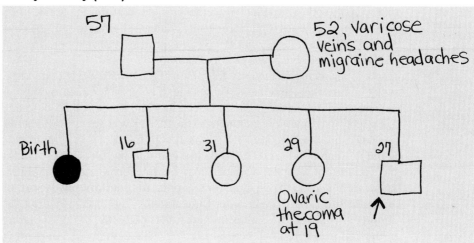

Review of Systems

In this section of the patient note, make a short review of systems (ROS). You can write it as a note or make a list of systems (e.g., respiratory, renal, neurological, etc.). Use your own criteria depending on the encounter you have. For CSA purposes, you have limited time. You will not be able to perform a complete or extensive ROS during the CSA exam. The format that you use will depend on the time available that you have to complete your notes. Remember, not all the information on the ROS will necessarily be pertinent to every case. Make the pertinent questioning of this part of the medical history as you perform the physical exam. Follow the same order as the physical examination format described in Figure 3–1. You can use a list of systems to describe your notes (e.g., cardiovascular, gastrointestinal, musculoskeletal). The ROS can be obtained during the physical exam. Try not to repeat symptomatology from the HPI.

The following example is a quick review of systems:

Review of Systems (Gen, Ob/Gyn, P)

HEENT and Neck: No alterations referred on direct questioning.
Chest: Grade 7 chest pain +, palpitations + and dyspnea to mild exercises and orthopnea.
Nocturnal paroxysmal dyspnea +, rheumatic fever antecedent +.
Respiratory: Unremarkable.
Renal/GU: Normal.
Extremities: Legs with bilateral edema grade 4.
Other: Normal.

ROS (Gen, Ob/Gyn, P)

Respiratory: No SOB, cough; unremarkable
Cardiac: No chest pain, dyspnea, orthopnea, palpitations, MI or murmurs.
GI: Vomiting 3x, no diarrhea, liver and gall bladder disease.
Renal: Nocturia 1x nightly without hesitancy, dribbling, or retention. No previous UTIs or renal calculi.
GU: No testicular mass, urethral discharge, or sexual difficulties.
Other: Unremarkable.

PHYSICAL EXAMINATION

This is the most important complementary part of the medical history. During the CSA exam, you need to be oriented to the problem that the SP dictates. You must be able to show your abilities to perform appropriate, well-oriented physical exam maneuvers, as well as communicate with the SP in a professional manner. The question you face is *How complete should the physical examination be?*

As in real clinical situations, the physical examination will depend on the chief complaint of the patient and the available time. It is very important to orient your physical examination maneuvers as well as the questioning. As explained before, do not forget to ask appropriate questions pertinent to the ROS as you are performing the physical exam.

Stay calm, organize your questions in your mind, and start the physical examination at the head and end on the feet. Before you start the physical examination, you should have an idea of what the diagnosis may be. In every anatomical approach, use the pertinent sequence of examination; for example, **inspection, palpation, percussion,** and **auscultation** is the correct order for examining the thorax, but not for examining the abdomen. Perform physical exam maneuvers correctly, trying to finding positive signs. In the CSA exam, you will be evaluated on what maneuvers you perform and how you perform them. When you are writing your patient notes, mention significant positive and negative signs. Make sure to speak clearly, always explaining to the SP what you will do before you proceed with any maneuver. Make appropriate eye contact, and use all equipment (e.g., table extension, gowns, ophthalmoscopes). Wash your hands before you examine the patient.

The following review of the physical examination and writing notes is for CSA purposes only. If you need more information, you can refer to any textbook on this matter.

General Examination

The general examination (GE) survey permits you to obtain an overview of the general state of the patient's health without focusing on a particular organ or system. During the first encounter and during the medical history, note how the patient looks (external habitus) as well as his gait, motor activity, personal hygiene, facial expression, speech, and any other obvious abnormalities. Individualize your notes depending on the case presented to you. Document the weight (W) and height (H) if you consider them pertinent; *vital signs* are documented as temperature (T), blood pressure (BP), *pulse* (P), and respirations (R), as appears on the doorway information sheet. You can reexamine any vital signs, but remember to only do this if it is necessary. Measuring the blood pressure can take you a few minutes, and you only have a total of 15 minutes to examine a patient during the CSA exam! For practical purposes, avoid double checking vital signs; just copy them on your notes as they appear on the doorway information sheet. Try to be precise and concise in this part of the note. You can summarize this information in one or two lines, according to the clinical situation of the SP.

See the following examples:

General Examination (Gen, Ob/Gyn)

Mildly ill appearing, no apparent distress observed.
T: 39.5°C, BP: 130/85 mm Hg, P: 100/min, R: 28/min.

GE (P)

An apparent normal full-term male newborn.
T: 39° C, BP: 65/50 mm Hg, P: 140/min, R: 30 res/min.
Somatic growth: H: 50 cm, W: 3070 g, head circumference: 36 cm, chest circumference: 32 cm.

General

Mildly disoriented, general aspect well.
BP 140/80, T 38°C, R 25/min, P 95/min.

Head, Eyes, Ears, Nose, and Throat

This part of the clinical exam includes the evaluation of the head, eyes, ears, nose, and throat, also known as HEENT. (You can also abbreviate ENT when you are referring only to the ear, nose, and throat.)

HEAD

Examine the head, scalp, skull, and facial musculature. Note any abnormality through inspection or palpation, skin color changes, masses or tumors, etc. If a neurologic deficit is detected, examine the correspondent cranial nerves (see Chapter 5). Remember to transluminate the patient's sinuses if you suspect sinusitis on the patient. Some experts think this maneuver does not help in the detection of sinusitis; however, you can perform it.

EYES

When you examine the eyes, observe the external eye, eyelids, pupillary size, shape, reactivity to light, extraocular muscle movement (EOM), visual acuity and visual fields (see Chapter 5). Perform a **visual acuity test** as explained in Chapter 5.

The signs and symptoms are very important on the eye assessment. Visual disturbances need an ophthalmologic evaluation. Burning and itching complaints are commonly seen by the generalist, and they may be caused by infections or minor trauma due to foreign bodies. If a foreign body is the problem, it is very important to document what kind of material might be involved. For example, contaminated material constitutes an emergency due to the risks of a corneal ulceration developing. Red eye is a common problem that needs an appropriate diagnosis. Some eye problems are obvious on only the clinical examination and are sufficient for the diagnosis; in other cases, specialist evaluation is mandatory. The differential diagnosis of red eye is showed is Table 3–1.

Diabetic retinopathy is the leading cause of blindness in the world, so it is mandatory to explore a fundal examination in all diabetic patients and more so in those with long-standing diabetes (i.e., more than 10 years with the disease). When you examine a diabetic patient, look for hemorrhages, exudates, and soft and hard neovascularizations in disc or elsewhere.

Glaucoma is the second leading cause of blindness in the United States. Glaucoma is often asymptomatic until the disease is well advanced or when the patient has decreased visual acuity field (i.e., tubular visual field).

Patients with glaucoma may present with complaints of perceiving **halos around lights** due to corneal edema and/or when the intraocular pressure is higher than 40 mm Hg. Acute closure angle glaucoma is an emergency and is manifested by a red painful eye, usually monocular, with progressive decreased vision and increased size pupil (approximately 6 mm).

EARS

Inspect the auricles and bilateral alignment, palpate the pre-, post-, and infrauriculary nodes, and perform a **quick acuity test** by occluding the tragus separately. If indicated by history, test the patient's capacity to hear whispered sound (normally it can be heard from 0.7 to 1.0 m away) and the wristwatch sound (possible to hear at 0.75 m) or by making a sound by rubbing the fingers together. More detailed auditory acuity examination includes the studies of the air and bone conduction using a tuning fork of 128 Hz and performing the Rinne test and Weber test (see Chapter 5).

Perform an otoscopic examination. Observe the external ear canals, and look for signs of inflammation on the inner skin or foreign bodies. Observe the tympanic membrane and note all normal and abnormal anatomic features of the drum (Figure 3–3).

NOSE

Observe the external aspect of the nose, palpate the septum, and use an anterior rhinoscopy (Thudichum speculum) or otoscope (without the disposable cone) to ob-

TABLE 3–1. Differential Diagnosis of Red Eye

Differential Diagnosis	Diagnostic Workup
1. Conjunctivitis (e.g., viral, bacterial, allergic)	1. Tonometry (measure of the ocular pressure)
2. Corneal injury	2. Gonioscopy
3. Foreign body	3. Sterile fluorescein strip + Wood lamp
4. Acute glaucoma	
5. Endophthalmitis	

Tympanic membrane

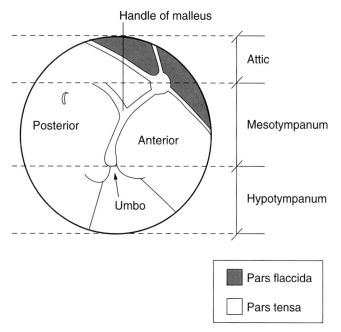

FIGURE 3–3. Anatomic features of the tympanic membrane.

serve the nasal septum and the inferior turbinate mucosa. Note any abnormal presence of polyps or papillomata. Finally, if indicated by history, assess the expiratory and inspiratory nasal airflow.

THROAT

First, observe the patient's face, expression, facial symmetries, deformities, and look for any lumps and bumps. Observe the lips. Ask the patient to open his mouth, and then inspect the buccal mucosa, gums, and teeth. Place special attention in periodontal hygiene and indicate the patient to remove any dentures if he/she wears ones; observe the tonsils, tell the patient to say "aahh", and observe the soft palate motion. Then, use a tongue depressor during this procedure to test the gag reflex if you consider this pertinent (see Chapter 5).

Sore throat is a common complaint, accounting for more than 10% of all office visits to the primary care practitioner. Throat examination must be followed by neck palpation to look for lymphadenopathy. Table 3–2 provides the general differential diagnosis of sore throat. Always order laboratory tests as indicated by history. There is controversy about when to culture an inflamed throat. Clinical features suggestive of group A β-hemolytic streptococcal pharyngitis includes fever greater than 38°C, anterior tender cervical adenopathy, lack of cough, and presence of pharyngea tonsillar exudate. Patients with mononucleosis may have marked lymphadenopathy, shaggy white-purple tonsillar exudate and hepatosplenomegaly. The typical patient is a young adult (15 to 30 years of age) who complains of sore throat and mild abdominal fullness sensation; the patient may be jaundice and may have close contact to someone with the same symptoms. Other infections may be due to viruses, bacteria, etc. *Neisseria gonorrheae* may be suspected in particular sexual practices. Diphtheria is uncommon today, but can be suspected by the presence of characteristic gray pseudomembrane and in alcoholic patients.

See the following general example of writing notes for HEENT:

TABLE 3–2. Differential Diagnosis of Sore Throat

Differential Diagnosis	Diagnostic Workup
1. Laryngitis	1. Throat culture[†]
2. Pharyngitis	2. CBC
3. Tonsillitis	3. Antistreptolysin O or rapid strep screen test[‡]
4. Epiglottitis	4. Monospot test[‡] (Heterophil agglutination test) or anti-EBV titer[§]
5. Infectious mononucleosis[*]	5. Peripheral blood smear (atypical lympho cytes)[//]
	6. LFT, including AST, ALT, AKP, and bilirubin (total and direct)
	7. CMV titers

ALT = alanine aminotransferase; AKP = alkaline phosphatase; AST = aspartate aminotransferase; CBC = complete blood count; CMV = cytomegalovirus; EBV = Epstein Barr virus; LFT = liver function tests.

[*]Acute disease due to EBV is characterized by malaise, fever, sore throat, and lymphadenopathy. Possible complications include hepatitis, myocarditis, neuropathy, and encephalitis.

[†]In patients with positive history of rheumatic fever or exposure to it.

[‡]Test for office use. They use streptococcal antigens from throat swabs. In general, these are less sensitive and more expensive than throat cultures.

[§]If negative, consider ordering CMV titers.

[//]Characteristic of mononucleosis, but also seen in CMV infections, toxoplasmosis, viral hepatitis, and rubella.

HEENT (Gen, Ob/Gyn) *(Extended format)*

Head: Normocephalic and free of visible lesions. Facial musculature revealed normal movement and adequate animation. Facial expression was consistent with and indicative of perceived pain.

Eyes: Ocular movements were normal. Conjunctivae clear without abnormalities.

Ear, nose, and throat: Pinnae were normal to inspection bilaterally. Ear canals showed no abnormalities on inspection. Nasal septum showed no deviation. Tongue was midline and normal movement of the soft palate was noted. There was no deficit on phonation.

HEENT (Gen, Ob/Gyn, P)

Conjunctivae clear without abnormalities or signs of infection.

Funduscopic exam; mild arteriolar narrowing without signs of exudates or arteriolar venous nicking.

Ear canal, tympanic membranes normal.

Oropharynx moderate injected retropharyngeal mucosa, without exudate.

HEENT (Gen)

Normocephalic free of visible lesions, visual acuity: RE 20/20 and LE 20/40, conjunctivae clear, pupillary reflexes present and normal. ENT without alteration.

Neck

For this portion of the physical examination, concentrate on inspection, palpation, and auscultation.

INSPECTION

Observe the neck from different angles, and observe any enlargement of the thyroid gland. Note the characteristics of the jugular veins by inspecting the jugular venous pulses. The neck veins can be viewed as manometers attached to the right atrium. By measuring the vertical height of the veins above the right atrium, it is possible to estimate the central venous pressure (CVP), which is an indirect reflection of right ventricular function. Note the highest point of oscillation or vein collapse of the internal jugular veins, which are relatively more difficult to see; and note the external jugular vein, which is relatively easier to see. Normally, when the patient is standing or sitting upright, the jugular veins are collapsed; when the patient is lying flat, they are completely filled. If the patient lies supine at approximate 45° (i.e., normal examining position), the point at which the jugular vein pulsation becomes visible is usually just above the clavicle.

To examine the patient, proceed as follows:

1. The patient should be placed at 30° to 45° of elevation.
2. Identify the highest point at which the pulsations of the jugular veins can be seen.
3. Identify the sternal angle (manubriosternal angle). By the use of centimeter ruler in vertical position, identify the intersecting point at 90° with a horizontal reference ruler or folded paper at the level of jugular veins' collapse (Figure 3–4).
4. Read the distance in cm above the sternal angle. Document the angle of the bed position and the jugular vein distention (JVD) in centimeters.

Because the sternal angle is about 5 cm from the right atrium (regardless of the elevation angle), the CVP can be estimated by adding 5 cm to the measurement. Some reference values and their correlation with the vertical height obtained in centimeters and the approximate pressure values are important to know (Table 3–3). Table 3–4 shows some differential diagnoses depending on the CVP.

Finally, when continuing the neck exam, ask the patient to swallow saliva or a small amount of water and observe the normal upward and downward movements as the pharyngeal muscles contract.

PALPATION

Palpate the lymph nodes along the body of the sternocleidomastoid muscle and lateral to the trachea and the anterior body of the trapezii. Finally, palpate the supraclavicular nodes; always remember to palpate the left supraclavicular nodes bilaterally. A palpable left supraclavicular node is known as **Virchow node.** Its presence alerts you to the possibility of gastrointestinal (GI) cancer. Palpate the thyroid gland, and note any abnormality in the texture (e.g., irregularities in the lobes, presence of nodules, enlargements and deep fixation) [Table 3–5]. In Plummer disease, one or more nodular areas

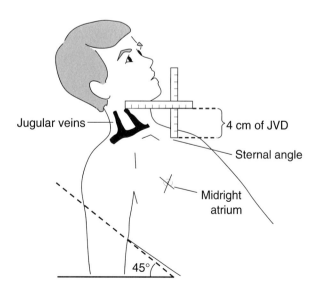

FIGURE 3–4. Estimating central venous pressure (CVP) during clinical examination. The zero blood pressure is in the right atrium. For conventional purposes, the zero point corresponds to the sternal angle.

TABLE 3–3. Determining Central Venous Pressure (CVP)

Height Above Sternal Angle (cm)	CVP	
	(cm H$_2$O approx.)	(mm Hg approx.)
1	6	4.4
2	7	5.0
3	8	5.8
4	9	6.6
5	10	7.4
6	11	8.0
7	12	8.8

Shaded area represents normal values. Normal CVP = 2 to 8 mm Hg.

are usually felt. In general, when hyperthyroidism is suspected, examine the moisture and temperature of the skin and note any exophthalmus, pretibial myxedema, and the reflexes. Palpate the carotid pulses.

AUSCULTATION

Auscultate the carotid arteries and the thyroid gland, noting any bruits. In Graves disease, the enlargement of the thyroid gland is uniform, and a bruit may be heard over the gland. Carotid auscultation is important in patients who are elderly, who are smokers, and who are diabetic or hypertensive, because of their risk for cerebrovascular disease.

The following are examples of medical notes for neck examination:

Neck (*Gen, Ob/Gyn, P*)

Supple without bruit, thyroid gland normal.

Neck (*Gen, Ob/Gyn, P*)

Single thyroid nodule (1 × 0.5 cm) noted on the right side; painless, soft, with regular borders and nonmobile. Cervical nodes negative; no bruits detected.

Neck (*Gen*)

JVD pulse 5 cm above the sternal angle at head (bed elevation of 45 degrees). No bruits or nodules were detected.

Chest

The correct order to perform the physical examination of the chest is **inspection, palpation, percussion,** and **auscultation.**

TABLE 3–4. Differential Diagnosis of Increased and Decreased Central Venous Pressure (CVP)

Increased CVP	Decreased CVP
Cardiac failure	Hypovolemia
Cardiac tamponade	
Excessive fluids	
Right ventricular failure	
Tricuspid insufficiency	

TABLE 3-5. Diseases of the Thyroid Gland

	Hyperthyroidism	Hypothyroidism	Thyroid Nodules	Thyroid Cancer	Thyroiditis
Etiology	Graves disease,* autoimmune by TSI immunoglobulins that activate the TSH receptor Toxic multinodular goiter Toxic adenoma Transient (postpartum silent thyroiditis, subacute thyroiditis, iodine induced) Thyroiditis Medication: levothyroxine, amiodarone	Hashimoto disease Lymphocytic thyroiditis Iatrogenic (thyroidectomy or radioactive iodine therapy) Medications: lithium, amiodarone, iodine Postpartum Subacute Thyroiditis	True adenomas Cysts Colloid nodules Hemorrhagic necrotic tissue Thyroid cancer	Types: papillar, follicular, medullary, anaplastic and metastatic Risk factors: neck radiation, hereditary (medullary cancer)	Acute: bacterial and viral Subacute: Known as Quervain disease, viral, Rickettsias Chronic: Hashimoto disease, autoimmune thyroiditis, such as silent, and postpartum
Clinical Manifestations	Hyperthyroidism symptoms (heat intolerance, weight loss, weakness, palpitations) Proptosis,* pretibial myxedema*	Hypothyroidism symptoms (cold intolerance, fatigue, somnolence, constipation)	Painless thyroid nodule Euthyroidism (except in toxic adenoma)	Painless thyroid nodule Euthyroidism (in most cases)	Thyroid gland becomes enlarged, tender, firm, pain radiating to ears or neck in acute and subacute cases. Initially may develop hypothyroidism symptoms and later hyperthyroidism.
Differential Diagnosis	1. Thyroiditis 2. Factitious hyperthyroidism 3. Anxiety disorders 4. Caffeine intake 5. Pheochromocytoma 6. Drugs (amphetamines, cocaine)	1. Primary and secondary hypothyroidism 2. Obesity 3. Depression	1. True adenoma 2. Thyroid cyst 3. Colloid nodule 4. Thyroid cancer 5. Hemorrhagic necrotic tissue	1. Follicular adenoma 2. Multinodular goiter 3. Colloid nodule 4. Thyroid cyst 5. Parathyroid mass 6. Neck metastasis	1. Graves disease 2. Toxic multinodular goiter 3. Toxic adenoma 4. Thyroiditis 5. Overmedication

continued

TABLE 3–5. Diseases of the Thyroid Gland *Continued*

Hyperthyroidism	Hypothyroidism	Thyroid Nodules	Thyroid Cancer	Thyroiditis
Diagnostic Workup 1. TSH: Expected results ($\downarrow$) 2. T_4: Expected results ($\uparrow$) 3. T3RU†† Expected results ($\uparrow$) 4. ECG 5. I-131 uptake: Expected results ($\downarrow$ in thyroiditis, $\uparrow$ in Graves and MNG, normal or $\uparrow$ in toxic nodule)	1. TSH: Expected results ($\uparrow$) 2. T_4: Expected results ($\downarrow$) If TSH is not increased, secondary hypothyroidism is the diagnosis; then study other pituitary hormones.	1. Fine-needle aspiration 2. Radionuclide thyroid scanning: Appears as "hot" in toxic adenoma and toxic MNG 3. Ultrasound 4. Computed tomography	1. Fine-needle aspiration 2. Ultrasound 3. Radionuclide thyroid scanning: cancer appears as "cold" on scan studies 4. TSH, T_4 5. CBC	1. TSH: Expected results ($\downarrow$) 2. T4: Expected results ($\uparrow$) 3. 24-hr RAIU: Expected results ($\downarrow$) 4. ESR: Expected results ($\uparrow$)

24 hr RAIU = 24-hour radionucleotide iodine uptake; CBC = complete blood count; ECG = electrocardiogram; ESR = erythrocyte sedimentation rate; T_4 = thyroxine; TSH = thyroid-stimulating hormone; TSI = thyroid-stimulating immunoglobulins.

* Characteristic only of Graves disease, not from other causes of hyperthyroidism.

†Indicates the plasma thyroxine-binding globulin (TBG). When TBG is decreased the T3RU is high and vice versa.

INSPECTION

Inspect the anterior, posterior, and lateral sides of the thoracic cage. During this initial step, note the presence of any chest wall deformities, such as barrel chest, pectum excavatum (tunnel chest) and pectum carinatum (pigeon chest). Note any operative scars. Observe the spine and note any deformities, such as kyphosis and scoliosis. Observe the breathing movements, and note any irregularities in frequency and rate; observe the equal motion of the chest. Pay special attention to patterns of breathing, such as Kussmaul, Cheyne-Stokes, and Biot breathing (Table 3–6).

Also observe the use of accessory muscles during the inspiratory effort. Note the patient's conversation during the clinical exam, paying special attention if the patient tolerates the lying down position.

Do not forget the two classic types of chronic obstructive pulmonary disease (COPD) patients. The **pink puffers** are characteristic because no cyanosis is noted, they are relatively elderly (i.e., older than 60 years), thin, usually do not present cough or expectoration. Further studies in these patients reveal that they have a predominant emphysema component, hypocapnia, and mild increase in airway resistance. The **blue bloaters** have the tendency to be cyanotic from hypoxia and bloated from right side heart failure (HF). They predominantly have a chronic bronchitic pattern more common in young age individuals, and they experience chronic cough, expectoration, and rhonchi.

Finally, continue with the clinical exam of the patient in supine position, noting the cardiac area. Note the heart's apical impulses, which are easier to observe in thin individuals and especially in the semi-Fowler position.

PALPATION

This part of the physical examination can be divided into two categories: palpation of the respiratory system and palpation of the heart.

Palpation of the Respiratory System

Start by palpating gently over the bones and on the cartilages. Pay special attention to any local tenderness. Note the presence of air in the subcutaneous tissues (surgical emphysema). Palpate thoroughly, and always ask the SP to guide you where he feels the complaint. Perform the following maneuvers:

Vocal fremitus. Place your palms on the thorax surface and then ask the patient to say different words or numbers, such as *13, 98,* and so forth. Remember that the passage of air in the normal lung is due to a specific consistency of the lung tissue and thus normal vibration sounds are transmitted to the chest surface. Any alteration on this normal characteristic, such as a mass consolidation, lobar pneumonia, or fluid-filled pleural space, will alter the transmission of sound in the vocal fremitus. For practice, first start recognizing the normal sensation on the normal lung; then you will notice the difference when you see an abnormal case. In general, the sound will be *increased* in consolidation (e.g., tumors, lobar pneumonia), *decreased* if there is air (pneumothorax), air/fluid levels (pleural effusion), or pleural thickening between the lung and the chest wall.

Vocal resonance is the same test as vocal fremitus, but it is performed by placing the stethoscope on the thorax. (For more information, see auscultation section).

Chest expansion is examined by placing both hands on the anterior thorax and the posterior surfaces of the thoracic cage and noting the chest movements. The thorax movements need to be symmetric in both hemithorax.

Respiratory excursion is assessed by placing the palms of your hands and thumbs symmetrically in both hemithorax at the same time, on the level of the eleventh ribs on the posterior area, and then on the anterior surface to the sides along each costal margin. Then ask the SP to breathe deeply. Observe the movement of your hands over the skin on the thoracic cage: normal movements are symmetric during the chest expansion (inspiration) and during the passive re-

TABLE 3–6. Patterns of Respiration

Type	Characteristic	Pattern
Normal respiration	Undulating symmetric pattern with sporadic increases of the peak flow of ventilation. Normal respiratory rate is 8 to 16 breaths/min.	
Tachypnea	Same pattern as normal respiration, but increased in frequency. Associated with diverse respiratory diseases that cause impairment in the V/Q*, pleuritic pain, restrictive lung disease. Respiratory rate > 16 breaths/min.	
Bradypnea	Same pattern as normal respiration, but decreased in frequency. Caused by drug-induced depression, increased cranial pressure. Respiratory rate < 8 breaths/min.	
Kussmaul breathing	Characterized by deep-sighing respirations as the patient tries to excrete CO_2. Characteristic in patients with metabolic acidosis from renal failure, DKA, aspirin overdose, anxiety. The area affected is in the midbrain or pons.	
Cheyne-Stokes	Also known as "periodic," or "cyclic" respiration. Characterized by waxing and waning respirations, depth over a minute or from deep to almost no breathing. It is caused by failure of the central respiratory control to respond adequately to the changes in the CO_2 and is seen in HF, uremia, brain damage. It may constitute a normal pattern in children and in aging patients during sleep.	Hyperpnea / Apnea
Biot breathing	Known as "ataxic breathing," it is characterized by an unpredictable irregularity. It can be a breaking shallow or deep pattern, then may stop and then continue. Its presence indicates a lesion in the medulla or brain.	
Obstructive breathing	Seen in severe COPD and asthma, it is due to increased airway resistance, causing a stopping and then continues with subsequent breathings.	

COPD = chronic obstructive pulmonary disease; DKA = diabetic ketoacidosis; HF = heart failure.
*Indicates the alveolar ventilation [V] versus the pulmonary blood flow [Q]; normal optimal ratio is approximately 1.

duction or expiration movements. Pay special attention to any abnormality in the respiratory movements. Alterations can be less movement in one side due to pleural effusion, lung collapse, pneumothorax, and pneumonia. A bilateral stopping movement due to pain is seen in pleuritis. Decreased movements in both sides are seen in generalized lung fibrosis and in chest wall problems, such as ankylosing spondylitis.

Palpation of the Heart

After observing the cardiac apical impulses, place the patient in the lying position at 45°. Place your hand on patient's chest (cardiac area) and note the point of maximal impulse (PMI), palpated at the fifth intercostal space and midclavicular line. The PMI are displaced by cardiomegaly, pregnancy, or other chest wall deformities. See Table 3–7 for associated diagnoses and characteristics.

PERCUSSION

For study purposes, this part of the physical examination is divided into percussion of the respiratory system and percussion of the cardiovascular system.

Percussion of the Respiratory System

The main purpose is to detect the **resonance** (hollowness) or **dullness** of the chest. First, be familiar with the normal percussion sound of the thoracic cavity—that is, the normal resonance of the lungs, the dullness of the liver, the tympanic sound of the gastric bubble.

Percussion of the Heart

Carefully percuss the heart area and delineate it, noting any abnormal findings. Pay special attention to any dullness or increase in the cardiac silhouette, which may indicate an increased cardiac size.

AUSCULTATION

For study purposes, this section of the clinical exam is divided into auscultation of the respiratory system and auscultation of the heart.

TABLE 3–7. Findings on Heart Palpation

Increased Force of the Apex	Decreased Force of the Apex	Thrill	Displaced Apex Beat
Meaning			
Increased cardiac output	Decreased cardiac output due to ventricular muscle damage	It is a palpable murmur	Apex beat is felt on different place.
Association			
Hyperthyroidism	Cardiomyopathy	Mitral insufficiency	Pregnancy: Beat felt upward
Fever	Myocardial infarction	Aortic stenosis	and directed to the left
Pregnancy		Ventricular septal defect	side
Anemia			RVH: Beat felt close to the
Anxiety			left sternal border
			Dextrocardia*: Beat felt on
			the right side

RVH = right ventricular hypertrophy.
*Very rare condition

Auscultation of the Respiratory System

The normal breath sounds heard over the normal lungs are two types: the **vesicular breath sounds** and the **bronchial breath sounds.** The abnormal breath sounds often are called **added sounds,** and these can be classified as **crackles, wheezes, stridor,** and **rubs.**

The vesicular breath sounds are produced in the small airways. They are transmitted through the airways and then attenuated by the lung structure through which they pass. The bronchial breathing sound is produced in the large airways, and is transmitted more or less unchanged through the lung tissue. The transmission of this sound is increased when the lung tissue itself acts as a solid mass, a good conductor for the wave sounds transmitting it from the origin site (central airway) to the skin (stethoscope bell). Those characteristics are like the vocal fremitus or vocal resonance. If a tumor is obstructing the central airway, there will not be transmission of sound, and then no bronchial breathing will be heard. The following are descriptions of abnormal, or added, sounds:

CRACKLES (Table 3–8). These are produced by air passage through the large bronchi that impacts with the secretions on it. They may be described as **fine crackles** that occur elsewhere in the lung tissue and are caused by bronchiectasis, pneumonia, pulmonary edema, and so forth. This sound is very similar to the sound produced by rolling the hair close to the ears.

WHEEZES are produced by the narrowing of the airway from any cause (e.g., asthma, COPD). If you suspect asthma in a patient and you believe that he or she has a severe attack (e.g., respiration > 28 bpm, heart rate > or = 110/min), you might check the presence or absence of pulsus paradoxus to confirm your diagnosis. Check the blood pressure, and see if it decreases by 10 mm Hg or more on deep inspiration. In an otherwise healthy patient, the BP changes are less than 5 mm Hg.

STRIDOR is better heard without a stethoscope and close to the patient's mouth. This sound indicates an obstruction or narrowing of the larynx, trachea, or main bronchi. For example, it is heard in epiglottitis.

RUBS are caused by inflammation of the pleural surfaces due to pneumonia, pulmonary embolism (PE), and so forth. They frequently are associated with pain on deep inspiration.

The reduction on vesicular breath sounds can be expected in severely obstructed airways (e.g., in asthma), emphysema, or in obstruction by a mass or tumor. The breath sounds are markedly reduced in emphysema, pneumothorax, over a particular bullae, pleural effusion, and pleural thickening. In general, any alteration between the lung and the chest wall will cause reduction in the breath sounds. It is important to mention some symptoms that are directly related to the respiratory system, such as cough.

Cough is a common complaint that you may encounter in a routine practice as well as on the CSA exam. This is a nonspecific symptom that may be produced by several factors that cause irritation on the tracheobronchial tree. Common causes can be infections, toxic substances, and neoplasms. Cough may be accompanied by other symptoms in lung diseases.

The differential diagnosis is wide, but depending on the medical history and physical findings, it can be narrowed. Table 3–9 provides a general differential diagnosis of cough. Not every examination or diagnostic workup is necessary. The overall assessment determines which tests are necessary for each patient; use your own criteria. If you have a patient/SP with systemic and cough symptoms that suggest that he has tuberculosis (TB) and you believe that he is a candidate for chemoprophylaxis, be prepared to discuss with him the possibility of it if a patient's skin test becomes positive. See Table 3–10 for diagnostic results criteria on PPD and prophylaxis indications.

Auscultation of the Heart

This is one of the best areas for a clinician to analyze and relate directly to the physiology and pathophysiology of the cardiac vascular system. It is not easy to detect small

TABLE 3–8. Abnormal Patterns on Respiratory System Examination

	Expansion/ Excursion	Vocal Fremitus	Percussion	Auscultation	Characteristics
Pleural Effusion	Decreased on affected side	Decreased if fluid compresses the lung; egophony; whispered pectoriloquy	Decreased; stony dullness	Breath sounds absent or markedly reduced	Caused by the presence of pleural transudate, exudate, blood, pus, or lymph; the mediastinum may be displaced away from the affected hemithorax
Atelectasia	Decreased on the affected side	Decreased; pectoriloquy may be heard	Normal or decreased	Breath sounds decreased; sometimes bronchial sounds are heard	Caused by bronch bronchial carcinoma, foreign body, infections, tuberculosis, bronchiectasias; the mediastinum may be displaced toward the lesion
Consolidation	Decreased	Increased	Decreased; dull to percussion	Breath sounds bronchial; whispering pectoriloquy; crackles	Caused by infections (e.g., *Streptococcus pneumoniae, Mycoplasma pneumoniae, Hemophilus influenzae*), aspiration, radiation
Pneumothorax	Decreased on the affected side	Decreased	Hyperresonant or normal	Decreased or absent	The affected hemithorax is at a higher pressure and tends to displace the mediastinum the opposite side; common causes include iatrogenic, unknown causes, apical blebs; infections)
Lung Fibrosis	Equally diminished	Normal	Normal	Decreased with crackles occasionally	The lungs are stiff; expansion reduced; common causes include cryptogenic fibrosing alveolitis, sarcoidosis, toxins)
Chronic Airflow Limitation	Equally diminished	Decreased or normal	Hyperresonant	Decreased vesicular sounds, added wheezes and crackles	This term involves COPD and asthma; mediastinum are central

COPD = chronic obstructive pulmonary disease.

TABLE 3–9. **Differential Diagnosis of Cough**

Differential Diagnosis	Diagnostic Workup
1. Rhinitis (postnasal drip)	1. CXR
2. Laryngitis	2. CBC
3. Pharyngitis	3. Sputum examination (Gram, KOH, acid-fast bacilli, cytology)[‡]
4. Bronchitis	4. Cultures (sputum, blood)
5. Pneumonia	5. PFT
6. Asthma	6. PPD
7. TB	7. Sweat test
8. COPD*	8. ABG
9. Malignancy	
10. Cystic fibrosis[†]	

ABG = arterial blood gases; CBC = complete blood count; COPD = chronic obstructive pulmonary disease; CXR = chest x-ray; PFT = pulmonary function test; PPD = purified protein derivative; TB = tuberculosis.
*Suspected in patients with chronic cough who have a positive history for smoking.
[†]Suspected in pediatric patients with multiple onsets of pneumonia, especially those caused by *Pseudomonas aeruginosa*.
[‡]If sputum production exists. Pertinent laboratory with other past medical history information or other important risk factors, such as smoking, TB exposure, travel exposure.

abnormalities on the heart sounds, even for the experienced clinician. There are several diagnostic tools to assess the heart. Before discussing cardiac auscultation, let us review how to use the chestpiece of the stethoscope. There are two types of stethoscopes, one with both bell and diaphragm and another with only a diaphragm. Normally, the bell is used to listen to low-frequency sounds, such as the S_3 and S_4 heart sounds, mitral stenosis, and blood pressure. The diaphragm is useful to listen to high-frequency sounds, such as lung and bowel sounds, mitral or aortic insufficiencies, and the S_2 heart sound.

TABLE 3–10. **PPD Indications and Diagnostic Criteria**

	Positive PPD Criteria		
5 mm	10 mm	15 mm	Indicated To (Isoniazid = INH 300 mg PO qd)
HIV infection	Immigrants from high prevalence countries (Asia, Africa, Latin America)	Any individual not in a high prevalence group	History of untreated TB or positive CXR
Defect on cell immunity			All skin reactors younger than age 35
Positive CXR with apical cavities	Homeless persons, prisoners		Changes from negative PPD to positive PPD within two years, regardless of age
Contacts of known causes	Nursing home residents		Positive factors regardless of age and at risk develop diseases, including those with AIDS, diabetes, ESRD, malignancy
	High-risk minorities (blacks, Hispanics)		
	Intravenous drug users		

CXR = chest x-ray; ESRD = end-stage renal disease; PPD = purified protein derivative; TB = tuberculosis.
(Adapted with permission from Ewald GA, Hackenzib C: *The Washington Manual,* 28th ed. New York: Little, Brown, 1995, p 322.)

TABLE 3–11. Heart Sounds

Heart Sound	Characteristics
S_1	Normal sound caused by the closure of the atrioventricular valves; this is a low-frequency sound that occurs just after the onset of ventricular contraction
S_2	Normal sound caused by the closure of the semilunar valves; it is a high frequency sound
S_3	This is a low-frequency sound caused by the rapid passive filling of the left ventricle. It is seen in heart failure and in young healthy athletes. It sometimes indicates a pathology in individuals older than age 40; it is also known as the "ventricular gallop."
S_4	Caused by atrial contraction; seen in the elderly due to a diminished compliance of the left ventricle; also seen in HTN and in CHF (caused by increase in the turbulence of the injected blood from the left atrium to the left ventricle). Pathologic sound known as "ventricular gallop."

CHF = congestive heart failure; HTN = hypertension.

See Table 3–11 for a description of heart sounds. In diaphragm-only stethoscopes, you can alternate both characteristics by alternating from the bell mode to diaphragm mode. For bell mode, just make a contact with the diaphragm on the skin very lightly; to use on a diaphragm mode, press the chestpiece firmly over the skin.

To auscultate the heart, start by auscultating at the base of the heart (aortic and pulmonic areas) using the diaphragm and then the bell on the specified areas according to Figure 3–5. Normally, S_2 is louder than S_1 at the aortic and pulmonic areas. Examine these areas and then proceed sequentially to examine the fifth left intercostal space, fifth left intercostal space medial to the midclavicular line, tricuspid area, and mitral areas, respectively. Pay attention to any abnormality and concentrate on describing the following parameters:

Heart rate. Confirm the heart rate posted on the doorway information sheet if you consider this pertinent.

Rhythm. Describe if it is regular or irregular.

Splitting. Concentrate on the S_2 sound at the pulmonic and aortic areas (Figure 3–6). Ask the patient/SP to breathe quietly, slowly and steadily.

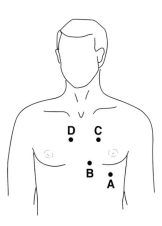

FIGURE 3–5. Heart auscultatory areas. **A)** Apex: good for hearing S_1 sound and murmurs from mitral valve. **B)** Lower left sternal border: good for hearing aortic reflux and tricuspid reflux. **C)** Upper left sternal border: good for hearing s_2 sound, pulmonary valve murmur, and ventricular septal defect. **D)** Upper right sternal border: good for hearing left ventricular murmurs (aortic stenosis).

FIGURE 3–6. S_2 splitting. During normal inspiration, the large vessels in the lung dilate; then the right ventricular output increases and the blood expelled is stored momentarily in the pulmonary arteries until expiration occurs. When expiration occurs, the blood flow reaches the left ventricle. In summary, splitting is accentuated by inspiration and usually disappears on expiration.

Location. Describe where the murmur is maximal.

Radiation. Examine the patient's neck and surrounding chest area. Note where the murmur radiates. For example, mitral murmurs radiates to the left axillae.

Other abnormal sounds can occur during the ejection phase (e.g., systolic clicks) or during the diastole (e.g., S_3, S_4, opening snap), including:

EJECTION CLICKS.   This is a high-frequency sound that follows shortly after the S_1. It is characteristic of pulmonary valve stenosis (pulmonic area). It also occurs in aortic valve disease and dilation of the aorta (aortic area).

OPENINGS SNAPS.   This is the diastolic sound that occurs during opening of the stenotic valve; it is best heard on the left of the sternum.

MIDSYSTOLIC CLICK is associated with mitral valve prolapse and may be accompanied with late systolic murmur.

MURMURS are sounds produced by the increase on the turbulent flow that occurs by the passage of blood through anatomic defect. Both systolic and diastolic murmurs can be described as early, mid, and late. Also, systolic murmurs that are heard throughout the systole are called pansystolic or holosystolic. Late diastolic murmurs may be called presystolic murmurs. It is very important to know how to grade murmurs. If you have a patient with a murmur, you must describe the grade of the murmur in your notes. The **grading/intensity** of murmurs are denoted on a scale from 1 to 6:

Grade 1: Difficult to hear

Grade 2: A quiet murmur, but audible with stethoscope

Grade 3: Easy to hear with stethoscope

Grade 4: Loud, obvious murmur; a thrill can be palpated

Grade 5: Very loud, heard not only on the precordium

Grade 6: Heard without stethoscope

Innocent murmur is a term used for murmurs in children and in young adults or athletes. They are characterized by being quiet (normally less than grade 3) and by not being related to ventricular hypertrophy or other heart sounds. Pulses, chest x-rays, and ECG are normal. An innocent murmur is best heard at the left sternal edge.

It is very important to make a clinical correlation of the patient. You are not expected to make a clinical diagnosis based only on the auscultation. The doorway information sheet and the general medical history from the SP are important information that give you a broad idea of several possible diagnoses. Remember, be prepared to answer an SP's questions about possible diagnoses and prognosis. Never give false reassurance to a patient; be sincere and professional.

Heart disease can be classified by the patient's symptoms and by following the New York Heart Association Functional Disability Grading System. This classification serves to quantify the limitation on activity of cardiac patients.

Class I: No limitation of physical activity. Ordinary physical activity does not cause fatigue, dyspnea, or anginal pain.

Class II: Slight limitation with mild to moderate activity (e.g., walking more than 2 blocks), but no symptoms at rest.

Class III: Marked limitation of physical activity. Comfortable at rest, but less than ordinary activity (e.g., walking less than 2 blocks) cause symptoms (e.g., dyspnea, pain).

Class IV: Symptoms at rest or with minimal activity, and symptoms of frank congestive heart failure.

The most common heart symptoms of heart disease are dyspnea, chest pain, palpitations, and syncope. None of these are pathognomonic of cardiac disease and its interpretation depends on the entire clinical picture. Chest pain is a common complaint and their presence announces multiple problems on different systems, such as musculoskeletal, respiratory, cardiac, and gastrointestinal systems. The most common cause of acute chest pain related to cardiac problem is ischemia. Table 3–12 lists a differential diagnosis of chest pain.

Dyspnea may be a sign of cardiac disease and indicate an elevated left atrial and pulmonary venous pressure or fluid overload. Dyspnea may also be caused by pulmonary disease. Cardiac dyspnea should be quantified by the amount of activity that precipitates it (see the New York Heart Association classification). Table 3–13 lists a differential diagnosis of dyspnea. Other terms to describe this symptom include **orthopnea** and **nocturnal paroxysmal dyspnea.** Orthopnea is a dyspnea that occurs in recumbency, and the nocturnal paroxysmal dyspnea is an acute shortness of breath (SOB) episode that awakens the patient at night, occurs 30 minutes to 2 hours after going to bed, and is relieved by sitting or standing up. Ask the patient the number of pillows that he or she uses to relieve his or her symptoms to sleep well at night. Note any edema in patients with heart failure, and do not forget to examine his or her legs. One way to document signs of cardiac edema is to measure and document the patient's weight during the physical exam if previous weight is known.

Palpitations are another symptom that may indicate cardiac disease. Palpitations are an awareness of the heart beating irregularly, rapidly, or unusually forcefully within the chest. Palpitations can be a normal phenomena that occur in athletes or in normal individuals; it is often associated with caffeine intake. Palpitations alone may be a symptom of diverse problems.

When palpitations are due to cardiac arrhythmia, they may be accompanied with syncope and light-headedness. It is important to make an appropriate analysis of this symptom. Questions about rhythmicity, or episodic skips or thump (by ectopic beats), can give clues about the underlying problem. Ask the patient: *How do you feel your car-*

TABLE 3–12. Differential Diagnosis of Chest Pain

Differential Diagnosis (as indicated by history)	Diagnostic Workup
1. MI	1. CXR
2. Angor pectoris/angina	2. ECG
3. Aortic dissection	3. CK-MB or troponin I or troponin T
4. Costochondritis	4. Electrolytes
5. Pericarditis	5. CBC
6. Pericardial effusion	6. V/Q SCAN
7. Pulmonary embolism	7. ABG
8. GERD	9. Echocardiography
9. Symptomatic diffuse esophageal spasm	10. Esophagus pH monitoring
10. Anxiety	11. Barium swallow

ABG = arterial blood gases; CBC = complete blood count; CK-MB = creatine kinase, myocardial bound; ECG = electrocardiogram; GERD = gastroesophageal reflux disease; MI = myocardial infarction; V/Q scan = ventilation perfusion scan.

TABLE 3–13. **Differential Diagnosis of Dyspnea**

Differential Diagnosis	Diagnosis Workup
1. CHF (due to MI, HTN, cardiomyopathies, valvular disease, or arrhythmias)	1. ABG or pulse oximeter
2. Asthma	2. CXR
3. COPD	3. ECG
4. Pneumonia	4. CBC
5. Anemia	5. Electrolytes
6. Anxiety	6. BUN/Cr
7. Obesity	7. Echocardiography
8. Fluid overload (e.g., in CHF, renal insufficiency)	

ABG = arterial blood gases; BUN/Cr = blood urea nitrogen/creatinine; CBC = complete blood count; CHF = congestive heart failure; COPD = chronic obstructive pulmonary disease; CXR = chest x-ray; ECG = electrocardiogram; HTN = hypertension; MI = myocardial infarction.

diac rhythm? Is it regular or irregular? Other questions may help you distinguish between palpitations caused by sinus tachycardia from paroxysmal arrhythmia: *Did the palpitations settle down gradually? Or did they stop suddenly like turning off a switch?* Final distinguishing between these conditions depends on the patient's history, ECG, or continuous Holter monitoring. Remember, you need to consider a range of possible diagnoses (up to five). Table 3–14 lists a differential diagnosis of palpitations.

Syncope is an abrupt decrease in cerebral perfusion causing brief loss of consciousness (i.e., fainting). Fainting itself can be due to benign conditions. When syncope is the chief complaint, you must try to determine whether the cause is benign or if there is a life-threatening condition (e.g., ventricular arrhythmia). The differential diagnosis is wide, but there are some clinical clues that may help you determine the cause of syncope (e.g, the presence of aura in seizures, history of sudden raising from bed or chair in orthostatism, sudden loss of consciousness in arrhythmias). Table 3–15 provides a differential diagnosis of syncope.

Cardiovascular disease causes 1 million deaths yearly, and half of these are due to coronary artery disease (CAD). The mortality of CAD is higher in the United States than other industrialized countries. It is very important to document information about the patient's risk factors for CAD (Table 3–16). Prevention of risk factors can be primary or secondary. Primary prevention involves the intervention on the modifiable risk factors

TABLE 3–14. **Differential Diagnosis of Palpations**

Differential Diagnosis	Diagnostic Workup
1. Cardiac disease (arrhythmias, valvular diseases, bradycardia)	1. ECG
2. Thyrotoxicosis	2. Holter monitoring
3. Anemia	3. Electrolytes
4. Exercise	4. TSH, T_4
5. Anxiety	5. CBC
6. Pheochromocytoma*	6. Urinary catecholamines, metanephrine, VMA
7. Drugs (amphetamines, cocaine)	

CBC = complete blood count; ECG = electrocardiogram; T_4 = thyroxine; TSH = thyroid-stimulating hormone; VMA = vanillylmandelic acid.
*Rare tumors localize on the adrenal glands or anywhere on the sympathetic nervous chain that are characterized by attacks of palpitations, headaches, perspiration, and high blood pressure.

TABLE 3-15. Differential Diagnosis of Syncope

Differential Diagnosis	Diagnostic Workup
1. Vasodepressor syncope	1. ECG
2. Orthostatic hypotension	2. Holter monitoring
3. Exertional syncope	3. EEG
4. Cardiac arrhythmia	4. CT scan (head)
5. Anxiety	
6. Seizures	
7. Transient ischemic attack	
8. Other (carotid sinus syndrome, micturition and tussive syncopes)	

CT = computed tomograph; ECG = electrocardiogram; EEG = electroencephalogram.

before the onset of the disease. For example, for patients who smoke, encourage and counsel them to quit. Help them set a quit date, provide self-help materials, and set up follow-up visits to assess compliance. Secondary prevention involves the intervention after the onset of the disease.

Not all the information that you may include on any particular section of the medical note is strictly related to the anatomic region that you are describing or had explored. For example, describing the jugular venous and peripheral pulses are pertinent to mention on cardiovascular examination. Other organ or systems related to patient's main problem can be included.

See the following examples of medical notes about the chest exam:

Chest (Gen, Ob/Gyn)

Respiratory: Coarse breath sounds in the right lower field with diminishing of the vesicular sounds. Wheezes and crackles were present. No dullness was detected.
Cardiac: No JVD, PMI palpable on normal position. Regular rate and rhythm. Normal S_1 and S_2, without murmur or gallop. Pulses normal.

Chest (Gen)

Respiratory: Normal breath sounds in the upper lobes. Bilateral basal crackles on the lower lobes. No wheezes.
Cardiac: JVP 8 cm at 45°, rhythm irregular, normal S_1, S_2 with S_3. No murmurs. Pulses were decreased. Class III functional disability.

TABLE 3-16. Risk Factors for Coronary Artery Disease

Modifiable Risk Factors	Nonmodifiable Risk Factors
Cigarette smoking	Positive family history
Increased LDL and decreased HDL	Gender
Increased serum cholesterol	Age
Hypertension	
Diabetes mellitus	
Estrogen deficiency	
Inactivity	
Obesity	

HDL = high-density lipoprotein; LDL = low-density lipoprotein.

Chest (Gen, Ob/Gyn, P)

Respiratory: Normal breath movements were noted, no cyanosis. Vocal fremitus and respiratory excursion were normal. No dullness. Wheezes were heard bilaterally with diffuse crackles +.
Cardiac: Normal S_1, S_2, no murmurs, rubs or gallops.

Chest (Gen, Ob/Gyn, P)

Respiratory: Decreased movement on the right hemithorax. Decreased vocal fremitus, dullness on percussion. No breath sounds were detected on R. lower lobe.
Cardiac: Normal PMI. Normal S_1, S_2. No murmurs, no JVD.

Abdomen

The correct order to examine the abdomen is **inspection, auscultation, percussion, and palpation.** The medical history is the most important tool in the study of patients with GI problems. Always accompany the GI exam with the palpation of the supraclavicular nodes and axillary nodes. As mentioned, the presence of palpable left supraclavicular node (**Virchow node**) and left axillary node (**Irish node**) always alerts you to the possibility of GI cancer.

INSPECTION

Observe the skin and note the presence of any abnormality, such as rashes, purpura, or evident hernias. Identify surgical scars, and name them properly as shown in Figure 3–7. On thin individuals, you may notice the pulsation of the abdominal aorta on the midline above the umbilicus, and sometimes the periodic rippling movement of the peristaltic movement on intestinal obstruction. Note the gravidae striae in women as well as the purple striae in patients with Cushing syndrome. Ascitic patients may present with a typical globular abdomen. Examine the skin for the presence of:

> **Grey Turner sign** is a bluish discoloration of either flanks seen in pancreatitis.
> **Cullen sign** is a bluish discoloration seen on the periumbilical area in pancreatitis.
> **Caput medusa sign** is visible vascular veins observed around the umbilicus, seen in liver cirrhosis.

Always describe your findings by dividing the abdomen in four quadrants with imaginary lines that crosses at the umbilicus. Figure 3–8 shows you two types of abdominal divisions.

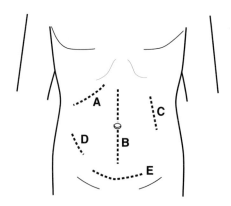

FIGURE 3–7. Surgical scars. **A)** Subcostal incision (cholecystectomy). **B)** Midline incision (laparotomy). **C)** Paramedian incision (cholecystectomy; no longer a commonly used incision). **D)** Rocky-Davis incision (appendectomy). **E)** Pfannenstiel incision (cesarean section).

AUSCULTATION

Start by placing the diaphragm of the stethoscope on the abdomen, and listen carefully to the bowel sounds. The normal bowel sounds (gurgling sounds) vary from 5 to 34/min in frequency, depending on the dynamic state of the bowel. The peristaltic sounds occur at 5 to 10 second intervals. An increase in frequency of bowel sounds can be caused by inflammation of the intestinal mucosa due to infections or inflammatory disorders, such as Crohn disease and ulcerative colitis. If your patient has hypertension, it is important to listen at the level of the epigastrium (2.5 cm above laterally to the umbilicus) to attempt to detect renal arterial bruits that can be caused by atherosclerotic disease, congenital renal artery disease, or fibromuscular hyperplasia.

Auscultate over the liver and the spleen areas. The presence of a soft bruit over the liver is always pathologic and may suggest either hepatitis or primary liver cell carcinoma. You may note a friction rub over the left hypochondrium in splenic infarction. Occasionally a rub over the spleen maybe heard, which may suggest an inflammation in the capsule.

PERCUSSION

This procedure is important for delineating the liver and spleen areas. Also, it is useful to identify the presence of ascitic fluid and solid or fluid-filled masses. You may alternate percussion with palpation. Start by percussing lightly in all four quadrants to determine the distribution of the gas in the abdomen. If you suspect ascites on the patient, place him or her in a supine position. The normal gas distribution on this position is to float above the ascitic fluid. As you percuss over the abdominal wall, you will notice the change of the percussion sound from tympanic or resonant to dull on the lateral sides. Mark the skin at the fluid gas level detected, then roll the patient to one lateral side and note the change of the position of the dullness and tympani. Mark the skin again (Figure 3–9).

PALPATION

This part of the abdominal examination can be divided into light and deep palpation.

Light Palpation

This procedure is particularly useful for detection of muscular resistance and abdominal tenderness and for exploration of superficial subcutaneous masses. Start by asking the patient to show you the area of pain or tenderness if abdominal pain is a presenting complaint. If the patient has a more localized pain, tell him to point to the area of

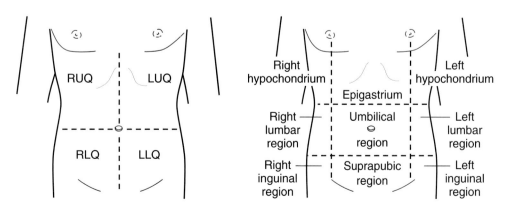

FIGURE 3–8. Abdominal divisions. RUQ = right upper quadrant; LUQ = left upper quadrant; RLQ = right lower quadrant; RUQ = right upper quadrant.

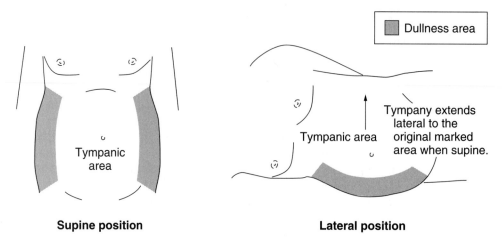

FIGURE 3–9. Patient with ascites.

pain with his finger. Begin light palpation in the area adjacent to tenderness site and then continuing to previously specified region (area of tenderness or pain).

Deep Palpation

Deep palpation is usually required to delineate the abdominal organs (liver, spleen, and kidneys) or other pathologic masses. Localize the anatomic area where the pain is referred by the patient, and cautiously make soft and light pressure. As you palpate the patient, try to imagine which organ is the cause of the problem. Initially the visceral pain (due to affection of the visceral peritoneum) will be referred to other regions distant from the original site of problem; as the inflammatory or irritative process continues, the parietal peritoneum become affected and the pain becomes somatic and then well-localized. As explained, the pain of appendicitis is initially referred in the epigastrium and/or in the periumbilical area, then may progress to be localized on the right lower quadrant (RLQ). If you have a patient with consistent symptoms of appendicitis, perform the following maneuvers:

REBOUND TEST   This maneuver can be performed by making a soft continuous pressure on the tender area followed by a sudden inadvertent removal of the hand. If this procedure exacerbates pain, it constitutes the **rebound sign.** Rebound sign is indicative of peritoneal inflammation, and it can be associated with appendicitis, tubal pregnancy, pelvic inflammatory disease, and ruptured ovarian follicle.

PSOAS TEST   For suspected appendicitis, have the patient lie down and then place your hand just above the patient's right knee; ask the patient to flex his leg at the hip against your resistance. An increase of pain on the RLQ constitutes the **Psoas sign** and is indicative of an inflamed appendix. This procedure is positive when the appendix is in retrocolic position adjacent to the iliopsoas muscle. Assess the patient by asking him if he can raise his legs while you oppose resistance over his knee.

OBTURADOR TEST   With the patient in the same position for the Psoas test, flex the same right thigh at the hip with the knee flexed (bent) and rotate internally or externally. A RLQ pain constitutes a positive **obturator sign.**

ROVSING SIGN   This test is positive when the patient complains of pain in RLQ at the moment of soft continuous compression of lower left quadrant (LLQ).

It is important to remember that all of these signs may be absent if the appendix is on anterior position or is wrapped in an inflammatory mass (phlegmon or omentum). The physical exam of a suspected patient with appendicitis can not be considered completed without performing a rectal or pelvic examination. (Do not forget to order this on your diagnostic work up plan in your patient notes.) Pain is also exacerbated on those maneuvers. If you find a mass during abdominal palpation (less probable), note the location, size, shape, consistency, adherence, tenderness, and so forth. Normally, the abdominal aorta is felt as a discrete pulsatile structure over the midline above the umbilicus; a large pulsatile mass on this localization may be indicative of aortic aneurysm. In 95% of cases, aortic aneurysms are asymptomatic; causes include atherosclerosis, trauma, infection, and syphilis. Evaluate by ultrasonography (USG), computed tomography (CT), magnetic resonance imaging (MRI), and aortogram. If you suspect an aortic aneurysm, check the peripheral pulses in the lower extremities; the extremities may look pallor, may feel cool, and the pulses may be diminished or unequal.

The liver and gall bladder must be explored by palpating the right upper quadrant (RUQ) using both hands or by the bimanual manner (placing one hand behind the patient and the other over the abdomen). Always talk with the patient, explaining every procedure that you are going to do. Looking to his head, proceed to delineate the upper and lower margin by palpation and percussion. The liver's normal sizes are 6 to 12 cms at the right midclavicular line and 4 to 8 at the midsternal line. Describe any abnormal characteristic, such as tenderness or nodularity.

Depending on your clinical suspicion, correlate your exam with other clinical data (e.g., jaundice tremors, upper GI bleeding, loss of hair on extremities, alteration on the mental status if you are suspecting liver cirrhosis, etc.). Ask the patient to take a deep breath as you try to palpate the lower margin of the liver and the gall bladder. The normal gall bladder is not palpated, but when obstructed and distended with bile, it can be detected on palpation. Determine the presence of **Murphy sign.** Murphy sign is characterized by the arrest of inspiratory effort as the examiner's hand contacts the inflamed gall bladder. The differential diagnoses of gallbladder disease is listed in Table 3–17.

There are many signs that can be related to liver and gall bladder disease. **Jaundice** is one of the most reliable and one of the first that the clinician frequently attributes. The differential diagnosis of jaundice is wide and may indicate more than liver diseases. Table 3–18 shows the differential diagnosis of jaundice.

Palpation of the spleen is similar to the liver, and under normal conditions the spleen will not be palpated.

The kidneys are not usually palpable, although on thin individuals it may be possible to palpate them. Deep bimanual palpation is required to explore the kidneys. The normal examination consists of sitting the patient on the examination table, placing your left hand over the costovertebral angle and striking on it with the ulnar surface of your right hand. Normally, no pain is perceived. On the inflamed kidney or in pyelonephritis, a costovertebral tenderness on the strike site will be referred.

The diagnosis of pyelonephritis sometimes is pathognomonic, especially on the adult patient. Urinary tract infections (UTI) can be classified as lower UTI (urethritis and cystitis) and upper UTIs (pyelonephritis). Lower UTI is characterized by dysuria, urgency, and frequency. On upper UTIs, there are costovertebral tenderness and fever, and there may be lower UTI symptoms. Table 3–19 lists special situations in UTI-suspected patients. Finally, keep in mind the differential diagnoses of renal masses and other associate pathologies in adults and children. Table 3–20 provides a differential diagnoses of renal masses.

The abdominal cavity has several organs, and there is no pathognomonic sign or symptom that is specific to each abdominal organ. Frequently, the signs and symptoms overlap each other, so it is very important to consider a wide possibility of diagnoses. Other disease factors, such as age, gender, and other risk factors, are very important to consider case by case. Abdominal pain is a common complaint that may be presented in an SP during the CSA exam.

The anatomic localization, quality, frequency, and form of pain presentation may

TABLE 3–17. Differential Diagnosis of Gall Bladder Disease

Cholelithiasis	Cholecystitis	Choledocholithiasis	Cholangitis
Clinical Signs and Symptoms			
50% of patients are asymptomatic, but may present with biliary colic*; RUQ pain or epigastric exacerbated by fatty meals.	Biliary colic RUQ tenderness and pain Fever Positive Murphy sign May be rebound and guarding	Biliary colic RUQ tenderness and pain Jaundice	1. Charcot triad: RUQ pain, fever, jaundice 2. Reynold pentad: RUQ pain, fever, jaundice, hypotension, mental confusion
Causes			
Calculi on the gall bladder without occlusion of the cystic duct	Calculi on the neck of the gall bladder or in the cystic duct	Calculi on the common bile duct (choledochus)	Calculi on the common bile duct plus infection in different stages (caused by *Escherichia coli, Klebsiella,* and *Strepto-coccus faecalis*) Acute ascending cholangitis Acute suppurative cholangitis
Workup Plan			
1. LFTs†: ALT, AST, AKP, direct and indirect bilirubin 2. Abdominal ultrasound 3. HIDA (if there is jaundice) 4. CBC	1. LFTs†: ALT, AST, AKP, direct and indirect bilirubin 2. Abdominal ultrasound 3. HIDA/PIPIDA 4. CBC	1. LFTs†: ALT, AST, AKP 2. Abdominal ultrasound 3. CT scan 4. ERCP 5. PTC 6. CBC	1. Before a full diagnostic work up, treat with IV fluids and ATB (ampi-cillin, gentamicin, metronidazole). 2. Surgical emergency: CBC, LFT, ultrasound, PTC/ERCP

AKP = alkaline phosphatase; ALT = alanine aminotransferase; AST = aspartate aminotransferase; CBC = complete blood count; CT = computed tomography; ERCP = endoscopic retrograde cholangiogram pancreatography; HIDA/PIPIDA = ra-dionucleotide biliary scan; PTC = percutaneous transhepatic cholangiogram; RUQ = right upper quadrant.
*Visceral pain that occurs in 75% of patients with gallstones or chronic cholecystitis. The pain usually follows a meal, begins abruptly, and is constant until it disappears (in a minute or hours).
†Never order LFTs like this. For CSA exam purposes, never order LFTs alone. Specify every test of the LFTs independently (e.g., ALT, AST, AKP, and so forth).

orient you toward the diagnosis. Knowing the origin of abdominal pain is useful to un-derstanding the differential diagnosis. As a general rule only, only three processes are capable of producing pain on the alimentary tract:

1. Pain caused by tension—e.g., powerful peristalsis caused by oxalic acid, in-fection, and so forth
2. Pain caused by ischemia—e.g., strangulation, obstruction, adhesion, volvulus
3. Pain caused by peritoneal inflammation (peritonitis)

Acute abdominal pain and colic type pain may be due to cholecystitis, ureteral stones, intestinal obstruction, and so forth.

Table 3–21 provides a differential diagnosis (by anatomical location) of acute ab-dominal pain. Only a minority of patients presenting with acute abdominal pain are found to have a problem that requires surgical treatment. It is very important to re-member that almost 50% of these patients have no identifiable causes of abdominal pain. Other conditions that do not require surgical treatment include gastroenteritis, pelvic inflammatory disease (PID), UTI, and ureteral stone. On any presented case with abdominal pain, it is important to consider the possibility of pneumonia; some basal lung pneumonias may cause a referred pain to the abdomen.

TABLE 3–18. Differential Diagnosis of Jaundice

Pre-hepatic Causes (Hemolytic Causes)	Hepatic Causes	Post-hepatic Causes
1. Sickle cell disease 2. Glucose-5-phosphate dehydrogenase (G5PD) deficiency 3. Spherocytosis 4. Autoimmune disorders 5. Drugs: methyldopa, antipsychotic drugs	1. Hepatitis A, B, C 2. Alcoholic hepatitis 3. Drug-induced hepatitis 4. Sarcoidosis 5. Disorders of bilirubin metabolism (Gilbert syndrome, Crigler Najjar syndrome, Rotor syndrome, Dubin Johnson syndrome, hemochromatosis, Wilson disease)	1. Gallstone disease 2. Common duct stricture 3. Primary sclerosing cholangitis 4. Gall bladder cancer 5. Common duct malignancies (Klatskin tumors) 6. Pancreatic cyst 7. Pancreatic cancer 8. Duodenal cancer
Diagnostic Workup	**Diagnostic Workup**	**Diagnostic Workup**
1. CBC plus peripheral smear 2. MCV 3. Cell solubility test or Hb electrophoresis 4. LFTs: ALT, AST, AKP, bilirubin 5. PT, PTT 6. Osmotic fragility test 7. G6PD levels 8. Direct Coombs test or direct antiglobulin test	1. CBC 2. LFTs: ALT, AST, AKP, bilirubin 3. PT, PTT 4. Hepatitis screen 5. Abdominal ultrasonogram	1. CBC 2. LFTs: ALT, AST, AKP, bilirubin 3. Abdominal ultrasonogram 4. HIDA scan 5. PTC 6. ERCP

AKP = alkaline phosphatase; ALT = alanine aminotransferase; AST = aspartate aminotransferase; CBC = complete blood count; ERCP = endoscopic retrograde cholangiogram pancreatography; HIDA = radionucleotide biliary scan; LFTs = liver function tests; MCV = mean cell volume; PT = prothrombin time; PTC = percutaneous transhepatic cholangiogram; PTT = partial thromboplastin time.

TABLE 3–19. Patient Profiles in Urinary Tract Infection (UTI)

Acute, Uncomplicated UTI in Young Women	Recurrent UTI in Young Women	UTI in Men Younger Than Age 50
Escherichia coli (80%) *Staphylococcus saprophyticus* bacteremia (15% to 20%)	Exogenous reinfection (90%) Relapse with original microbe	Does not necessarily indicate urologic tract abnormality. Uropathogenic strains can cause pyelonephritis. Risk factors include sexual partner with uropathogenic strain colonization, anal intercourse, and lack of circumcision.
Diagnostic Workup 1. Urinalysis 2. Urine culture 3. Blood culture	1. Urinalysis 2. Urine culture	1. Urinalysis 2. Urine culture

TABLE 3–20. Differential Diagnosis of Renal Masses

ADULTS		CHILDREN		
Renal Carcinoma	Polycystic Kidney Disease	Wilms Tumor	Neuroblastoma	Polycystic Kidney Disease
Clinical Features				
Abdominal mass, flank pain, hematuria, fever, fatigue, anemia	Flank mass, abdominal mass, proteinuria, hematuria, HTN, UTI	Abdominal mass; peak incidence < 5 years of age, abdominal pain, hematuria, HTN	Abdominal mass is the most common presentation; flank pain, HTN; other locations: thoracic, head/neck	Commonly diagnosed during infancy; oliguria, renal insufficiency, hepatomegaly
Causes				
Pipe and cigar smoking; known renal cell adenocarcinoma, Grawitz tumor, hypernephroma	Autosomal dominant disorder; out-pouchings may also occur in the liver, pancreas, and vascular tree	Neoplastic embryonal cell of the metanephros	Malignancy of the neural crest cells; second most common solid tumor in children	Autosomal recessive disorder; usually detected at birth
Diagnostic Workup Plan				
1. USG 2. CT/MRI 3. IVP 4. Nephrotomograms 5. Urinalysis 6. CBC 7. Electrolytes	1. USG 2. Urinalysis 3. ES 4. CBC 5. Electrolytes 6. Biopsy	1. USG 2. IVP 3. CT/MRI 4. Urinalysis	1. USG 2. Urinary markers: VMA, HVA 3. Serum markers: Neuron-specific enolase, ferritin, and LDH 4. Oncogene marker: N-myc oncogene	1. USG 2. Electrolytes 3. Urinalysis 4. CBC

CBC = complete blood count; CT = computed tomography; HVA = homovanillic acid; IVP = intravenous pyelogram; LDH = lactate dehydrogenase; MRI = magnetic resonance imaging; USG = ultrasonogram; VMA = vanillylmandelic acid.

The GI system is an important system that mandates special attention to symptoms. Common symptoms related to the GI system are dyspepsia, nausea and vomiting, diarrhea, dysphagia, hiccups, constipation and signs related to GI bleeding (e.g., hematemesis, hematochezia, and melena).

Dyspepsia is an imprecise term to describe an upper abdominal discomfort, such as epigastric tenderness, fullness sensation, bloating, early satiety, heartburn, or regurgitation. The differential diagnosis of dyspepsia is listed in Table 3–22. **Nausea** and **vomiting** are symptoms that may involve more than a GI system abnormality. Systemic illness (e.g., CNS disorders), side effects of medications, and some viral illnesses may cause nausea and vomiting. Also, nausea and vomiting are common symptoms of pregnancy. If intestinal obstruction is not suspected, common antiemetics and oral intake limited to clear fluids are helpful to control it.

Diarrhea can be classified as acute or chronic. The approach to a patient with diarrhea consists of trying to identify and treat the possible cause, control any fluid and electrolyte abnormality and, if indicated, use of antidiarrheal medications. Table 3–23 provides a classification and etiologic differential diagnosis of diarrhea.

Esophageal diseases are commonly manifested by dysphagia, odynophagia, or heartburn. **Dysphagia** is a difficulty in swallowing and is commonly described as a sticking sensation. **Odynophagia** is pain on swallowing. It is important to know if dysphagia is for solids or liquids. **Heartburn** is described as substernal burning sensation that radiates toward the mouth and is increased by bending forward. Table 3–24 provides a differential diagnosis of esophageal diseases.

TABLE 3–21. Differential Diagnosis of Acute Abdominal Pain

RUQ	RLQ	Epigastrium	Periumbilical	Hypogastric†	LUQ	LLQ
1. Acute cholecystitis 2. Kidney stone 3. Pancreatitis 5. UTI 6. Pneumonitis	1. Appendicitis 2. Urethral stone 3. Ruptured ectopic pregnancy 4. PID 5. UTI	1. PUD 2. Esophageal spasm 3. Acute pancreatitis 4. Appendicitis 5. Acute cholecystitis 6. MI	1. Appendicitis 2. Acute mesenteric ischemia 3. Ruptured aortic abdominal aneurysm 4. Acute intestinal obstruction	1. Ruptured ectopic pregnancy 2. Acute intestinal obstruction 3. PID	1. Ureteral stone 2. Splenic rupture‡	1. Ureteral stone 2. Acute diverticulitis 3. PID 4. UTI

Diagnostic Workup

RUQ	RLQ	Epigastrium	Periumbilical	Hypogastric†	LUQ	LLQ
1. Urinalysis 2. Abdominal ultrasound 3. IVP 4. Abdominal x-rays 5. CBC	1. Pelvic/rectal exam 2. Urinalysis 3. CBC 4. Abdominal x-rays 5. Abdominal ultrasound 6. CXR	1. Endoscopy 2. Serum amylase 3. CBC 4. Abdominal ultrasound 5. Abdominal x-rays	1. CBC 2. Abdominal x-rays* 3. Rectal exam 4. Guaiac test 5. Abdominal ultrasound	1. Pelvic/rectal exam 2. Pelvic/vaginal ultrasound 3. Abdominal x-rays 4. Guaiac test 5. CBC	1. Urinalysis 2. Abdominal ultrasound 3. Abdominal x-rays 4. CBC 5. IVP	1. Urinalysis 2. Abdominal ultrasound 3. Abdominal x-rays 4. CBC 5. IVP

CBC = complete blood count; CXR = chest x-ray; IVP = intravenous pyelogram; LLQ = left lower quadrant; LUQ = left upper quadrant; MI = myocardial infarction; PID = pelvic inflammatory disease; PUD = peptic ulcer disease; RLQ = right lower quadrant; RUQ = right upper quadrant; UTI = urinary tract infection.

*Abdominal plain radiographs in two positions (upright and decubitus) are very helpful in suspected causes of ileus and/or intestinal obstruction. Look for air-fluid interfaces.

†Also known as suprapubic

‡Very rare condition associated with previously diseased spleen. Worldwide, the most common cause is malaria, followed by infectious mononucleosis.

Hiccups are a sporadic and unremarkable symptom that generally does not mandate medical consultation. However, chronic, recurrent hiccups may indicate a severe condition that mandates further examination. Table 3–25 lists a differential diagnosis for hiccups.

Constipation is a common complaint that you may be presented with during the CSA exam. Constipation can have several causes, such as lack of exercise, medications (e.g., aluminium hydroxide, anticholinergics, iron supplements, narcotics, antihyper-

TABLE 3–22. Differential Diagnosis of Dyspepsia

Differential Diagnosis	Diagnostic Workup
1. GERD	1. Barium swallow and upper GI series
2. PUD	2. Acid reflux test
3. Gastroparesis	3. Endoscopy
4. Biliary tract disease	4. Serum amylase
5. Pancreatitis	5. Abdominal ultrasound
6. Gastritis	
7. Hiatal hernia	
8. Other (heart disease)	

GERD = gastroesophageal reflux disease; GI = gastrointestinal; PUD = peptic ulcer disease.

TABLE 3–23. Differential Diagnosis of Diarrhea

Differential Diagnosis		Diagnostic Workup
Acute diarrhea	**Chronic diarrhea**	
1. Infectious agents (viral, bacterial, parasitic)	1. Lactose intolerance	1. Stool cultures
2. Drugs (laxatives, antiacids, digitalis, quinine, colchicine, antibiotics*)	2. Pancreatic cholera syndrome‡	2. Fecal methylene blue for fecal leukocytes
3. Inflammatory bowel disease (can be chronic)	3. Irritable bowel syndrome	3. Stool ova and parasite examination
4. Zollinger-Ellison syndrome† (can be chronic)	4. Inflammatory bowel disease	4. Guaiac testing to detect occult blood
5. Whipple disease (can be chronic)	5. Diabetic neuropathy	5. Fecal Sudan staining to detect fat droplets
6. AIDS enteropathy	6. Postvagotomy or post-gastrectomy syndromes	6. Stool pH
7. Carcinoid syndrome (can be chronic)	7. Food allergy	7. Lower endoscopy
	8. Hyperthyroidism	

*Includes pseudomembranous colitis, which is associated with clindamycin. Most common in hospitalized patients.

†Zollinger-Ellison syndrome is direct result of the independent production of gastrin by a tumor arising on the pancreas or paraduodenal region.

‡This syndrome is characterized by watery diarrhea, hypokalemia, and achlorhydria. It is known as VIPoma, pancreatic cholera, or Verner-Morrison syndrome. VIP is a vasoactive intestinal peptide produced by a tumor of the non-beta cells of the pancreas.

tensives), or systemic diseases (e.g., hypothyroidism, diabetes, hypercalcemia). It is important to question the patient about the presence of tenesmus (pain during the defecation), which may indirectly cause constipation. Ask about and document any change in the pattern of stools, including consistency, thickness, or presence of blood. Colon cancer always needs to be considered.

Finally, it is very important to consider the evaluation of a patient with **GI bleeding.** Hemodynamically unstable patients are treated initially by maintaining an adequate circulatory volume, and their initial assessment is oriented initially toward monitoring the heart rate, blood pressure, urinary output, postural changes, and so forth. Nonacute GI bleeding can be evaluated in the office and can be classified as upper or lower GI bleeding, depending on the signs and symptoms.

TABLE 3–24. Differential Diagnosis of Esophageal Disease

Differential Diagnosis	Diagnostic Workup
1. Reflux esophagitis	1. Barium swallow and upper GI series
2. Scleroderma	2. Endoscopy with biopsy
3. Esophageal motor disorders	3. Acid reflux test
4. Symptomatic diffuse esophageal disease	4. Esophageal manometry
5. Achalasia	5. Scintigraphy
6. Esophageal rings	
7. Esophageal webs (Plummer-Vinson syndrome)	
8. Benign esophageal stricture	
9. Esophageal carcinoma	

*Abdominal plain radiographs in two positions (upright and decubitus) are very helpful in suspected causes of ileus and/or intestinal obstruction.

TABLE 3–25. Differential Diagnosis of Hiccups

Differential Diagnosis	Diagnostic Workup
Benign hiccups	
1. Gastric distention	1. Neurologic exam
2. Sudden temperature change (e.g., drinking hot or cold liquids)	2. CBC
3. Alcohol ingestion	3. Electrolytes
4. Emotional state (e.g., excitement, stress, laughter)	4. BUN/Cr
	5. LFT: AST, ALT, bilirubin
	6. CXR
	7. Other: CT head scan, echocardiogram, bronchoscopy, endoscopy
Recurrent hiccups	
1. CNS neoplasms	
2. Metabolic: uremia, hypocalcemia, hyperventilation, electrolyte imbalance	
3. Irritation of the vagus or phrenic nerve	
4. Other causes	
HEENT: foreign body in ear	
Neck: goiter, neoplasm	
Thorax: pneumonia, empyema, neoplasm, MI, pericarditis, aneurysm, esophageal obstruction, reflux esophagitis	
Abdomen: subphrenic abscess, hepatomegaly, hepatitis, cholecystitis, gastric distention, cancer	

ALT = alanine aminotransferase; AST = aspartate aminotransferase; BUN/Cr = blood urea nitrogen/creatinine; CBC = complete blood count; CNS = central nervous system; CT = computed tomography; CXR = chest x-ray; HEENT = head, eyes, ears, nose, throat; LFT = liver function test; MI = myocardial infarction.

Upper GI bleeding may be suggested by the presence of **hematemesis** or **melena.** When hematemesis is referred, upper airway sources or hemoptysis must be ruled out. The approach to those patients depends on the patient's stability, the rate of blood loss, procedural availability, and local expertise. Lower GI bleeding can be referred as **hematochezia** or brisk blood in feces, or can be suggested during positive Guaiac test (i.e., hemoccult-positive stool test). Remember, this test may have false-positive results due to certain foods (e.g., broccoli, radishes, turnips, roast beef) and medications (e.g., Pepto-Bismol). A Guaiac test can be performed quickly in a routine office visit. Also, in the United States, there are kits that the patient can use to get his own samples of feces at home and then mail to physician's office. Table 3–26 lists the differential diagnosis of GI bleeding.

See the following examples of writing notes about the abdominal examination:

Abdomen (Gen, P)

Normal abdominal bowel sounds; soft, nontender, without hepatosplenomegaly.

Abdomen (Gen)

Abdominal bowel sounds absent. Tenderness on superficial palpation on lower right quadrant pain, rebound and guarding positive.

Abdomen (Gen)

4 cm Rocky-Davis incision on the R. inguinal region, well healed without signs of erythema, redness or discharge. Normal abdominal bowel sounds. Moderate diffuse tenderness, no hepatosplenomegaly.

TABLE 3–26. Differential Diagnosis of Gastrointestinal (GI) Bleeding

Differential Diagnosis	Diagnostic Workup
Acute GI Bleeding	
Immediate exact diagnosis not important; stabilization of patient is mandatory.	1. Crossmatching 2. CBC* 3. PT, PTT 4. Chemistries (electrolytes, renal function tests, glucose)
Upper GI Bleeding	
1. Duodenal ulcer 2. Gastric ulcer 3. Erosive gastritis 4. Esophageal ulcer 5. Angiodysplasia 6. Mallory Weis tear 7. Neoplasms	1. Esophagogastroduodenoscopy 2. Arteriography 3. Upper GI barium series† 4. Guaiac test† 5. CBC
Lower GI Bleeding	
1. Diverticulosis 2. Angiodysplasia 3. Neoplasms 4. Inflammatory bowel disease 5. Ischemic colitis 6. Infectious colitis	1. Rectal examination 2. Guaiac test 3. Arteriography§ 4. Technetium-99 red blood cell scanning// 5. Colonoscopy** 6. CBC

*CBC is a poor indicator of acute blood loss.

†It has no role if the institution has available endoscopy.

‡This test can be used as a screening tool to diagnose GI bleeding. It can be performed during the office visit or performed by the patient in home by the use of secure US mail approved kits.

§Detects arterial bleeding rates of 0.5 ml/min. Indicated if the patient is hemodynamically unstable due to a brisk bleed.

//Detects arterial bleeding rates of 0.1 ml/minute.

**Allows direct identification of the problem, is therapeutic (e.g., electrocautery) and diagnostic (i.e., biopsy). Also indicated if the arteriography and 99-Tc red blood cell scan was negative.

Abdomen (Gen)

Globular abdomen with old surgical scar on the midline. Hyperactive abdominal bowel sounds with metallic character. Moderate tenderness on the umbilical region. Marked tympani on percussion.

Abdomen (Gen)

Globular abdomen on inspection. Bowel sounds present but ↓ on intensity and frequency. Diffuse tenderness, central tympani, dullness on the sides.

Genitalia

Always remember that on the CSA, you are not allowed to perform a genital exam.

This section covers genitourinary disorders in adult men. Chapters 4 and 7 cover female and pediatric genitourinary disorders, respectively.

During the CSA, if you have an SP with symptoms related to the male genital area, obtain detailed information about the signs and symptoms. Think about a probable diagnoses and discuss with the SP what he might have. Remember that you can examine the inguinal area, especially palpation, if the clinical setting mandates it.

One important clinical setting that you may encounter during the CSA exam is the presentation of an older male with obstructive urinary symptoms. It is more probable that you will encounter an older man with hesitancy, poor stream, a sensation of incomplete bladder emptying after voiding, and nocturia rather than an SP with acute urinary retention symptoms with vesical distention. Be prepared to explain the importance of performing a rectal examination **(but don't perform it!).** If the clinical setting suggests, reassure him that he may have a benign prostatic hyperplasia (BPH); however, other conditions, such as UTI and prostatic cancer, need to be ruled out. Explain that BPH is a common problem of males, and its frequency increases with age. Table 3–27 provides a differential diagnosis of hesitancy.

The following medical notes are only an example, and those marked with an * reflect the type of examining that you are **not** allowed to perform during the CSA exam:

Genitourinary (Gen)

Inguinal canal and testes were normal; inspection was unremarkable.* On palpation of the suprapubic region, the bladder appears full and this maneuver stimulates micturition.

GU (Gen, P)

Positive urethral discharge. Two inguinal lymph nodes palpated bilaterally. Testes were normal.*

Genital (Gen, P)

Soft mass was palpated on the scrotum on the left side.* After reduction into the inguinal canal, no protrusion was noted after Valsalva maneuver.

Neurologic

This part of the clinical exam varies greatly. You can perform a quick neurologic screening test if the case presented to you does not mandate further examination. But if the SP has a neurologic problem, you need to perform an organized and complete neurologic exam (see Chapter 5). Remember, the neurologic exam is performed as part of the medical history depending on the clinical case (see Chapter 5).

Motor and sensory examinations are described briefly as follows:

Neurologic (Gen)

Alert, well oriented X 3. Cranial nerves normal. Motor 5/5. Sensory intact to pin, vibration, and proprioception. Deep tendon reflexes were 3/4. Plantar reflexes downgoing.

TABLE 3–27. Differential Diagnosis of Hesitancy

Differential Diagnosis	Diagnostic Workup
1. BPH	1. Rectal exam
2. Prostatic cancer	2. Urinalysis and culture
3. UTI	3. BUN/Cr
4. Bladder calculi	4. Transabdominal ultrasound*
	5. Prostate specific antigen
	6. Transrectal ultrasound†
	7. Urinary flow rates

BPH = benign prostatic hyperplasia; BUN/Cr = blood urea nitrogen/creatinine; UTI = urinary tract infection.
*This exam has replaced the intravenous pyelogram.
†Used to evaluate irregular prostate on rectal exam.

Neuro (Gen)

DTRS showed 2+ responses symmetrically. Gait was significantly impaired. Hypersensitivity to sharp stimulus was detected in the right C5/C6 dermatomes. Group by group motor exam revealed ↓ muscle strength (+4/+5) for the right wrist and finger flexors.

Neurologic (Gen)

Patient was alert, oriented × 3. Cranial nerves show asymmetry to movements on facial muscles on the right side (CN VII), loss of taste and hyperacusis. Motor 5/5. DTRs were 2/4. Plantar reflexes downgoing.

Musculoskeletal System

On the CSA, each part of the musculoskeletal (MSK) system does not need to be examined in every patient. Some patients may present with a localized complaint (e.g., shoulder pain) and you may only need to focus on that area. It is unnecessary to perform all the tests systematically to every patient; some patients may need only some maneuvers, others may need a more detailed exam, and others may only need some maneuvers in the context of a general clinical exam. Use your own criteria.

Learn how to describe properly the movements from different joints and extremities of the body. It is not the purpose of this book to include detailed information about MSK system, but some of the information about the maneuvers or particular problems will be discussed here.

One important thing to know is the acronym **RICE** (**R**est, **I**ce, **C**ompression, **E**levation). Most of the common injuries (e.g., knee or ankle sprains/strains) are treated with the RICE recommendations. Be prepared to explain to the SP these recommendations.

The MSK exam is performed basically with inspection and palpation, although percussion and auscultation may be used. Knowing how to properly execute MSK exam maneuvers is very useful, because an appropriate exam helps you formulate a differential diagnosis. None of the clinical exams are pathognomonic for one disease; keep in mind the possibilities regarding the diagnosis, especially during the CSA exam.

As a general rule, start from the head and end at the feet. It is very important to make a general inspection to try to find obvious problems, such as genu valgus or varus on the extremities. When you refer to a particular joint movement, it is important that you consider the normal anatomic position (Figure 3–10).

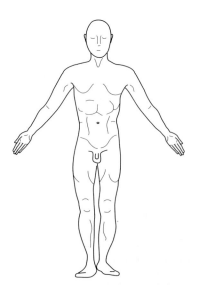

FIGURE 3–10. Anatomic position.

Finally, depending on the underlying cause and patient history, order appropriate tests. Consider x-rays if a deformity exists or a traumatic event occurred. If you suspect a rheumatologic problem, antinuclear antibody (ANA), erythrocyte sedimentation rate (ESR), and rheumatoid factor may serve as screening tests.

HEAD AND NECK

The movements of the neck are:

Flexion (anterior)
Extension (posterior)
Lateral movements to the right and left
Rotational

You can assess the patient by telling him to move his head forward and backward and to each side. Ask him to let you know when he feels stiffness or pain. Note any decrease in the range of motion.

Cervical Foraminal Compression Test. Place soft to moderate pressure with your hands over the patient's head and push downward. Ask him if he feels a referred pain on the neck, or if its radiates to the sides. Positive test may indicate a cervical disk disease, cervical spondylosis, cervical sprain, cervical strain with or without radiculalgia and herniated disc.

On your notes, you can write as follows:

Musculoskeletal (Gen, Ob/Gyn, P)

Pain and tenderness to palpation of the posterolateral neck, exacerbated by flexion, extension, rotation and lateral flexion movements.
Cervical Foraminal Compression Test was positive for localized posterior pain.

Musculoskeletal (Gen, Ob/Gyn, P)

Pain and tenderness to palpation of the posterior neck. Pain was exacerbated by lateral movement to right side only. Cervical foraminal compression test was positive bilaterally but increased on the right.

SPINE

The movements of the spine are:

Flexion (anterior, 75° to 90°)
Extension (posterior, 30 °)
Lateral bending
Rotation movements to the sides (right and left)

Assess by telling the patient to perform those movements; note any alteration or pain. Inspect the normal spine position or any alteration, such as syphosis and scoliosis. Palpate the paravertebral muscles, spinous process; note any tenderness, muscles spasm, pain, and trigger points. Then percuss or make soft strikes with your hand over the spine on different points.

Herniated intervertebral disks are most common between L5 and S1 or between L4 and L5; this may produce tenderness on palpation over the spinous process, over the intervertebral muscles, and over the joints. Sciatic pain also can be exacerbated by this maneuver. Other causes of pain include rheumatoid arthritis and ankylosing spondylitis. Remember that costovertebral angle tenderness may suggest kidney infection. Finally, during the examination, don't forget to ask the patient to cough. Sciatic pain is exacerbated by coughing.

On your notes, you can write as follows:

Back (Gen, Ob/Gyn, P)

Pain and tenderness to palpation in the middle and low back, exacerbated by flexion, extension, and lateral bending. Palpation was + for tenderness and pain over the L1-L4 spinous process and right lumbosacral tenderness.

Back (Gen, Ob/Gyn)

Pain and tenderness to palpation of the low back, exacerbated by flexion, extension, rotation, lateral flexion, and coughing.

SUPERIOR EXTREMITIES

It is very important to describe properly the movements of the different joints on the upper limbs. We will divide this review into examination of the shoulder, elbow, wrist, and hand.

Shoulder

This unique joint has several complex movements that differ from those of other joints. The general movements of the upper arm at the shoulder are:

Forward flexion from neutral position or 0° (arms down) to 180° (arms up)
Extension from 0° (arms down) to 50° (arms behind)
Abduction (0°)
Adduction (180°)
Internal and external rotation

Assess the patient by telling him to raise his arms, move them backward and forward, open them, and so forth. Note the presence of pain or limited range motion. Causes of pain in this area may include acromioclavicular joint bursitis, tendinitis, and capsulitis. Palpate the joint and trapezii muscles, and identify areas of pain, tenderness, associate myospasm, and trigger points.

Shoulder Depression Test. Make a soft continuous pressure with your hands over the patient's shoulder pushing downward. Ask him if he feels a referred pain on the neck or over the joint. A positive test may indicate a shoulder strain or sprain, traumatic injury of the shoulder, and cervical strain or sprain.

On your notes, you can write as follows:

Musculoskeletal (Gen, Ob/Gyn, P)

Pain and tenderness to palpation of the upper trapezii, with multiple trigger points detected in association with gross myospasm. Shoulder depression test was positive on the right.

Musculoskeletal (Gen, Ob/Gyn, P)

L. shoulder joint pain and tenderness exacerbated by flexion, extension, and abduction movements. Pain and tenderness to palpation of the left coracoid process was detected. Shoulder depression test was + on the L.

Elbow

The movements at the elbow are:

Flexion/extension
Supination/pronation

Assess the patient by observing the extension and flexion movements at the elbow. Supination and pronation can be examined by asking the patient to fist his hand as if he is holding a pencil between the fingers (Figure 3–11) and observing the movements. The normal range of movements are from 0° to 90° for supination and 0° to 90° for pronation.

Note any abnormality or difficulties during the movements. Common conditions that affect this joint are lateral and medial epicondylitis (also known as tennis elbow and golf elbow, respectively). The physical examination includes point tenderness over the involvement site exacerbated by flexion and extension of the wrist on movements against his resistance. The term *at* on your notes may have a particular meaning, indicating the joint in which the movement is performed.

On your notes, you can write as follows:

Extremities (Gen, Ob/Gyn, P)

Pain and tenderness on extension and flexion movements of the forearm at the elbow. Limited range of motion were noted at 30 degrees on extension. Supination/pronation was normal.

Extremities (Gen, Ob/Gyn, P)

Pain and tenderness on flexion/extension movements refereed to the medial epicondyle.

Ext (Gen, Ob/Gyn, P)

Limited range of motion on pronation of 50° at the elbow. Flexion and extension movements were normal.

Wrist

Starting with hands in the normal anatomical position, the wrist movements are (Figure 3–12):

Extension (hands to the back)
Flexion (hands to the front)
Radial deviation (lateral movement to the radius bone)
Ulnar deviation (lateral movement to the ulnar bone)

Note the presence of any abnormality during these movements, including pain, tenderness, or limited range of motion. Write your notes as follows:

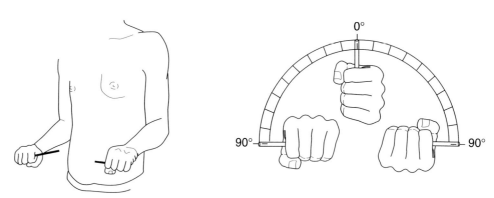

FIGURE 3–11. Supination–pronation and range movements of the elbow. Adapted with permission from Hoppenfield S: Physical Examination of the Spine and Extremities. Appleton-Century-Crofts, 1976 (Spanish edition).

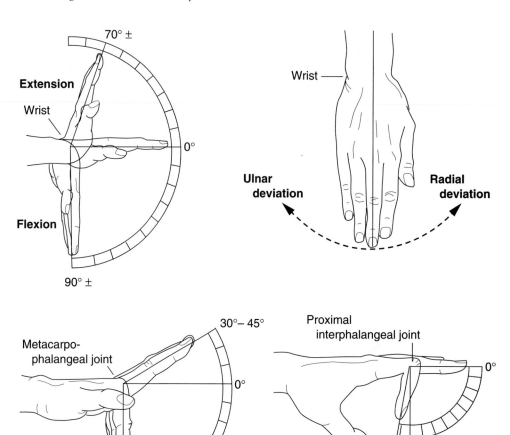

FIGURE 3–12. Hand and wrist movements. Adapted with permission from Hoppenfield S: Physical Examination of the Spine and Extremities. Appleton-Century-Crofts, 1976 (Spanish edition).

Ext (Gen, Ob/Gyn, P)

Pain and tenderness on flexion and extension movements of the hand at the wrist. No abnormalities on lateral movements.

Extremities (Gen, Ob/Gyn, P)

Pain on radial deviation movement of the hand at the wrist but not on ulnar deviation. Flexion/extension were normal.

Hand

The hand has several movements that need a detailed description, depending on the joint at which the movement is performed. The movements of the hand can be at the level of the wrist, at the metacarpophalangeal joint (MCP), proximal and distal inter-phalangeal joints (PIP and DIP), respectively (see figure 3–12).

Carpal tunnel syndrome is characterized by pain, tingling, and numbness over the palm of the hand and on the thumb, index, middle, and half part of the ringer fingers. The symptoms usually appear at night, and sometimes awake the patient. This problem is caused by an entrapment of the median nerve in the carpal tunnel. This nerve provides sensation in the half part of the palm and permits the pinch movement.

To examine a patient with these symptoms, perform the following tests:

Phalen Test. Hold the patient's hand in acute flexion at the wrist for 60 seconds. If numbness and/or tingling develop over the distribution of the median nerve innervation fingers, the sign is positive.

In conjunction with Phalen test, tap the median nerve at the wrist and note if the patient complains of tingling of the hand fingers **(Tinel sign).** Factors that are related to carpal tunnel syndrome include the repetitive usage of the hand and tendons (e.g., typing on a keyboard), trauma, infections, use of oral contraceptives, pregnancy, obesity, diabetes mellitus, hypothyroidism, gout, and rheumatoid arthritis. Differential diagnosis of this pathology includes cervical radiculopathy, ulnar neuropathy, transient ischemic attack (TIA), and diabetic neuropathy. The diagnostic tool to diagnose this pathology includes EMG studies and x-rays.

Finally, note any abnormality, such as pain, tenderness, or limited range motion, which may occur on examination of the hand joints.

See the following examples of writing medical notes:

Extremities (Gen, Ob/Gyn, P)

Pain on flexion and extension movements of the R. middle fingers at the MCP joint.

Extremities (Gen, Ob/Gyn, P)

Pain on flexion and extension of the index R. finger at the PIP joint.

Ext (Gen, Ob/Gyn, P)

Pain and tenderness on flexion and extension movements at the DIP joint.

Ext (Gen, Ob/Gyn)

No pain or tenderness on flexion and extension movements of the R. hand at the wrist. No abnormalities on lateral movements. Phalen's and Tinel's signs were positive on the R. hand.

INFERIOR EXTREMITIES

For CSA review purposes, this part of the physical examination can be divided into examination of the hip, knee, ankle, and feet.

Hip

The movements of the hip are (Figure 3–13):

Extended, on neutral position as on supine position or standing

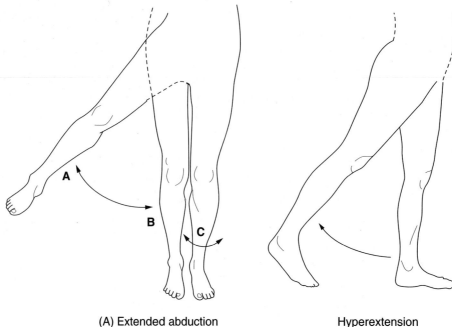

(A) Extended abduction
(B) Extended adduction
(C) Internal/external rotation

Hyperextension

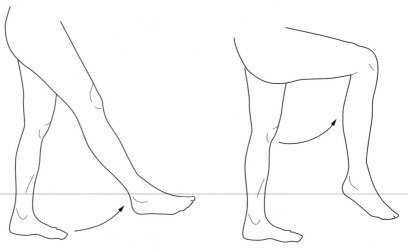

Flexion with knee straight

Flexion with knee flexed

FIGURE 3–13. Hip movements.

Hyperextension, back to neutral position
Flexion with the knee straight
Flexion with the knee flexed
Abduction
Adduction
Internal/external rotation

The flexion movements are examined with the patient in the supine position. The hyperextension, abduction/adduction, and internal/external rotation are examined with the patient in standing position. Review the following tests.

Straight Leg Raising Test (SLRT). With the patient in the supine position, flex the leg at the hip with the knee straight. Normally, the leg can be flexed to 90 degrees. The SLRT is positive if it produces back pain or sciatic pain that can be increased by dorsiflexing the foot. With sciatic pain, the pain is relieved by flexing the leg at the knee or by extending the leg at the hip. The differential diagnosis of low back pain is described on Table 3–28. Some clinical findings on this test may suggest a tentative diagnosis. These findings include:

Radiculopathy—the test elicits sciatic neuralgia on dorsiflexion of the foot with the leg flexed at the hip with the knee straight
L4-L5 herniation—the test exacerbates pain between 0° to 20°, this might indicate and herniated disc

Trendelenburg Test. Have the patient stand up, and have him use the wall or a chair for holding support. From behind the patient, observe him stand on one foot and lift the opposite knee above the level of his waist. Normally, this action causes an elevation of the gluteal fold along with the pelvis ipsilateral above that of the standing leg side. The Trendelenburg test is positive when the gluteal fold is lowered by raising the leg on the same side. The significance of this abnormality will include gluteal (abductor) insufficiency on the standing leg side. The differential diagnosis of this finding includes coxa vara, coxa valga, and congenital dislocation of the hip. The test must to be done bilaterally. Finally, note any abnormality, such as pain, tenderness, or limited range of motion.

See the following examples of writing medical notes:

Musculoskeletal (Gen, Ob/Gyn, P)

Straight raising leg test was negative bilaterally.

Musc/Back (Gen, Ob/Gyn)

SRLT was positive on the right at 45° for localized moderate back pain and on the left at 25°, exacerbating pain that radiates to the left thigh and buttock.

Musc/Back (Gen, Ob/Gyn)

SRLT was positive bilaterally for localize low back pain at 20° and 25° on the R. and L. respectively.

TABLE 3–28. Differential Diagnosis of Low Back Pain

Differential Diagnosis	Diagnostic Workup
1. Lumbar sprain (ligamentous affection)	1. Lumbar spine x-rays series (useful if antecedent of trauma exist)
2. Lumbar strain (muscular affection)	
3. Sciatica (radiculopathy)	2. CT/MRI lumbar scans
4. Lumbar disk herniation	3. EMG
5. Spinal stenosis (Pseudo if claudication exists)	4. ESR
	5. CBC
6. Spondylolisthesis	
7. Tumor, infection	

CBC = complete blood count; CT = computed tomography; EMG = electromyography; ESR = erythrocyte sedimentation rate; MRI = magnetic resonance imaging.

MSK/Back (Gen, Ob/Gyn, P)

Difficulty on abduction of the R. leg at the hip. SRLT was negative bilaterally. Trendelenburg test was positive to R. side.

Knee

The normal movements of the knee are flexion and extension. Sometimes anterior hyperextension may be found. Assess as for other joints, noting any abnormality. Auscultation may be helpful, especially when you try to hear a "click" referred by the patient. Examine the knee with the following tests.

Stability Knee Test. Key symptoms that indicate using this test are complaint that the knee "buckles" or "gives way." To perform this test, tell the patient to lie down and flex the knee to 80°. Stabilizes the foot by gently sitting on the examining table. Hold the leg with both hands below the knee, and then try to move backward and forward (Figure 3–14). Evaluate the results as follows:

Increased anterior mobility: Anterior cruciate ligament instability
Increased posterior mobility: Posterior cruciate ligament instability

---

McMurray Test. With the patient in the supine position, flex the leg at the hip with the knee bent (flexed) between 120° and 160° (Figure 3–15). Then with one hand, hold the patient's knee (thumb and index fingers on each side of the knee) and with the other hand hold and rotate laterally his foot. Ask the patient if he feels pain, tenderness, clicking, locking, or popping sensations inside his knee. At the same time, try to feel the click on your hand. The test is positive if you heard or palpate the click, which may be due to a medial meniscus displacement.

See the following examples of writing notes:

Extremities (Gen, Ob/Gyn, P)

No pain or tenderness was detected on knee flexion and extension movements. Stability knee test was positive for anterior instability. McMurray's test was negative.

Ext (Gen, Ob/Gyn, P)

Pain on extension of the knee was detected. Stability knee test was negative for instability but produced pain and tenderness. McMurray's test was positive on the inner side.

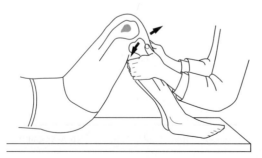

FIGURE 3–14. Stability knee test.

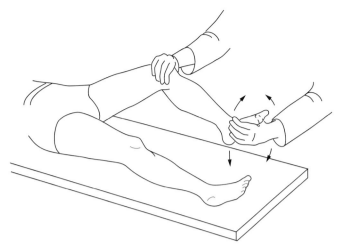

FIGURE 3–15. McMurray test. With the patient in the supine position, flex the leg at the hip with the knee bent (flexed). Then with one hand hold the patient's knee, and with the other hand hold and rotate laterally his foot.

Ankle and Foot

The movements of the foot at the ankle are:

Dorsiflexion or plantar extension
Plantar flexion (downgoing)
Inversion (inner movement)
Eversion (external movement)

Take note of the results on your examination and be prepared to compose the medical note. Common problems that involve this region are ankle sprains, which are frequently related to sports injuries. The varus inversion at the foot is the most common form. Ankle sprains are classified as follows:

Grade I: Mild injury
Grade II: Moderate injury
Grade III: Severe injury, which is characterized by excessive anterior motion of the foot on anterior applied force (positive test)

Review the following examples of written notes:

Extremities (Gen, Ob/Gyn, P)

Pain on inversion of the foot. Flexion, extension, eversion movements were normal.

Ext (Gen, Ob/Gyn, P)

Pain and tenderness on inversion movement of the R. foot. Anterior motion of the foot was noted.

DIFFERENTIAL DIAGNOSIS

It is impossible to explain in a single chapter how you should delineate and choose a diagnosis during the CSA exam. Each clinical encounter will have its own characteristics and diagnosis. Keep in mind that most patients do not go to a physician to obtain a diagnosis—they go to relieve their symptoms. Some patients may need an appropriate explanation of the problem to relieve his or her anxiety. It is very important to be prepared to explain to the patient what you think he or she has. Some patients are very concerned that they are going to die. Some patient with chest pain may be scared that they are having an MI! Be prepared to answer the patient's questions properly, not prematurely, during the interview, but always after completing the clinical exam. The development of hypothesis by a researcher is the equivalent of making a differential diagnosis by a physician. The differential diagnosis is confirmed by the clinical or laboratory diagnosis. Your overall clinical preparation gives you the necessary tools to choose appropriately what laboratory exams you need to order.

DIAGNOSTIC WORKUP

Learn how to summarize common laboratory results the way that it is done in the United States health care system (Figure 3–16). Normally, certain tests are performed routinely in every new admitted patient. These tests may include complete blood count (CBC), electrolytes, x-rays, electrocardiogram (ECG), and so forth. Americans use the standard stick figure in Figure 3–16 to communicate to another health professional the results of these tests. For example, you may hear or tell somebody that: CBC; WBC 12; H/H: 14 and 40; platelets, 15. Electrolytes: 140/5 (Na^+/K^+), 103/24 (Cl^-/Bicarbonate$^-$), 12/1.2 (BUN/Cr), 105 (glucose).

For CSA purposes, you need to **list up to five diagnostic tests** that the SP should have. Be explicit and precise. Use appropriate abbreviations and first-line tests. See the following examples writing notes and examples how to use the stick figures of CBC, electrolytes:

Diagnostic Workup Plan

1. EKG
2. Electrolytes
3. CXR
4. CBC
5. Troponin I

Diagnostic Workup Plan

1. Sinus x-rays series: Lateral skull x-rays, Cadwell and Waters
2. CBC with differential
3. Protein C

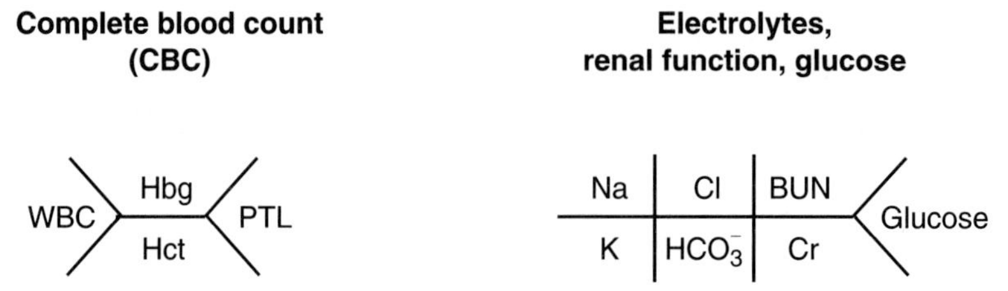

Complete blood count (CBC)	Electrolytes, renal function, glucose

WBC = White blood cell (x 10/μL)
Hbg = Hemoglobin (g/dl)
Hct = Hematocrit (ml/dl)
PTL = Platelets (x 10/μL)

Na = Sodium (mEq/L)
K = Potassium (mEq/L)
Cl = Chloride (mEq/L)
HCO_3 = Bicarbonate (mEq/L)
BUN = Blood urea nitrogen (mg/dl)
Cr = Creatinine (mg/dl)

FIGURE 3–16. Summarizing laboratory results.

Diagnostic Workup Plan

1. Stool ova/protozoa examination
2. Fecal methylene blue
3. Stool pH
4. CBC
5. Electrolytes

$$14.0 \big\rangle\!\!\frac{15}{45}\!\!\big\langle 190.0 \qquad \frac{140}{4.5}\bigg|\frac{102}{24}\bigg|\frac{20}{1.5}\big\rangle 105$$

4

Obstetrics and Gynecology: Writing Medical Notes and the Physical Examination

INTRODUCTION

Obstetrics and gynecology (Ob/Gyn) is a medical field in which it is necessary to obtain information from a patient in a very discrete form. The medical history, although similar to other histories, has particular differences. The correct use of Ob/Gyn terminology can give you an idea of a particular symptom that will also help you quantify it. Obviously, your approach to the patient in this medical field will depend largely on previous clinical experiences and rotations. Remember, during the CSA exam you are not expected to perform a pelvic exam. This chapter contains more information about obstetrics than gynecology, but gynecologic aspects are also discussed. The chapter begins with an introduction to the physiology of pregnancy, followed by a description of the most common terms used in an Ob/Gyn written note.

PHYSIOLOGY OF PREGNANCY

Pregnancy is a normal physiologic state, not a disease, that causes several changes in a woman's body. Pregnancy is divided into trimesters (Figure 4–1). The first trimester lasts from conception until 14 weeks of gestation; the second trimester is from 14 weeks until 28 weeks; and the third trimester is from 28 weeks until delivery. It is important to review some aspects of the normal and abnormal changes caused by pregnancy. These changes occur in all the body systems, but for the purposes of this book they are divided into general and local.

General Changes

SKIN

Hyperpigmentation of the skin appears during the first month of pregnancy and tends to disappear after delivery, although it may persist. Hyperpigmentation can appear on the face (known as cloasma), breasts, areola, abdomen (linea bruna), and genital area. Other changes include the presence of the gravid striae, which appears on the abdomen

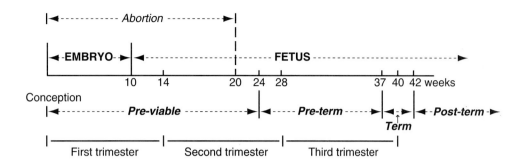

FIGURE 4–1. Chronology of pregnancy.

during the second trimester and spider telangiectasias, which may appear on the face, neck, arms, and thorax.

BREASTS

Starting in the second month, the breasts enlarge and become somewhat nodular to glandular as the ductal tissue increases. The nipple enlarges and becomes darker; colostrum can be expressed from the nipple after the 16th week of gestation until 3 or 4 days after delivery.

BASAL TEMPERATURE

There is an increase in basal temperature of 0.3°C to 0.6°C during the first trimester of pregnancy. Shortly after the 14th week, this starts to decrease slowly.

INCREASE IN MATERNAL WEIGHT

During pregnancy, a woman increases her weight by approximately 20% of her previous weight (approximately 10 to 12 kg or 22 to 29 lb). During the first trimester, maternal weight stays the same or may diminish due to vomiting (and therefore a loss of fluid). During the second trimester, weight gain can be 1200 g/month. During the third trimester, the weight increase is approximately 1500 g/month, but becomes less during the last 2 weeks of gestation. There should not be a weight increase of more than 500 g/week during the third trimester. If such an increase occurs, fluid retention/preeclampsia is suspected.

METABOLISM

Water

At the end of pregnancy, there is a water increase of 6000 ml that represent 50% of the overall increase in maternal weight.

Protein

During pregnancy a positive "nitrogen balance" occurs; 1000 g of protein are distributed as follows: 500 g to the fetus and placenta and 500 g to the maternal blood, the uterus, and the breasts.

Iron

Iron levels are decreased during pregnancy. The iron requirement is 800 mg (300 mg to the fetus and 500 to the mother). During the first half of pregnancy the iron requirements are supplied by the maternal reserves, but the requirements increase during the second part of the pregnancy. Normally, elemental iron (30 to 60 mg/day) should be given to supplement the diet. Remember, iron is also found in red meat, liver, green vegetables, whole grain cereal, dried fruits, and beans.

HEMATOLOGIC CHANGES

The blood volume increases 45% to 50%. The fraction that most increases is the plasma (70%) in relation to the hematocrit (30%). These nonproportional increases are the cause of the physiologic anemia that occurs during pregnancy. Pregnancy is also a hypercoagulable state. There is an increase in fibrinogen and factors VII through X; however, clotting and bleeding times do not change. The number of thromboembolic events during pregnancy are increased.

White Blood Cells

Physiologic leukocytosis appears with values between 11,000 and 16,000/μL, due principally to an increase of neutrophils.

Hemoglobin/Hematocrit

Both hemoglobin and hematocrit are lowered in a parallel form. In the 32nd to 35th weeks of gestation, hemoglobin (Hb) can decrease 11 g/100 mL and hematocrit (Hct) can decrease approximately 33%. There are no changes in the peripheral smear.

Platelets

Thrombocytosis occurs, with values increasing to 500,000 to 600,000/μL.

Total Protein

Total protein value is decreased, but the globulin fraction increases slightly. The albumin fraction is decreased. The normal albumin to globulin ratio is 1.35. This progressively decreases until reaching values of 1.0 or 0.8.

Total Lipids

Total lipids increase during the second half of pregnancy, reaching values of 1000 mg/100 mL (mean value, 700 mg/100 mL) in the 40th week of pregnancy. Cholesterol reaches its maximum value (300 mg/dL) in the 30th week.

Glucose

There is no alteration in glucose during pregnancy compared with the healthy, nonpregnant woman. However, diabetes can occur during pregnancy. The cause of glucosuria during pregnancy must be investigated. However, glucosuria does not necessarily indicate hyperglycemia, because glucosuria can be due to a lower renal threshold for glucose, which may be induced by a normal pregnancy. The levels of several hormones (progesterone, estrogen, cortisol, human placental lactogen) are elevated during pregnancy; together, they can have a diabetogenic effect.

MUSCULOSKELETAL SYSTEM

There is a normal change in the mother's posture due to a shift in the center of gravity. Consequently, there is lower back strain and lumbar lordosis. Softness of the ligaments also occurs throughout the body, causing an increase in ligament movements.

CARDIOVASCULAR SYSTEM

Because of the increase in uterine size, the heart and the point of maximal impulse (PMI) move to the fourth intercostal space away from the left breast line. There is also an increase in cardiac output and splitting of the S_1. Systolic murmurs in any of the auscultatory points are frequently heard. The murmurs are due to changes in the great vessels, the displacement of the heart, and the increase of the turbulent flow:

$\mathbf{Re = v \times D \times d/n,}$ where

Re = Reynolds units (a measure of turbulence)

v = velocity

D = diameter

d = density

n = viscosity, due to decreased blood viscosity by hemodilution

Blood pressure does not change during the first months of the pregnancy but can increase slightly during the last 2 months. Any significant increase in arterial blood pressure needs to be studied for the possible appearance of preeclampsia. Jugular vein pressure (JVP) and right atrium pressure do not change, but the venous pressure on the lower extremities progressively increases due to the cephalic compression of the fetus over the iliac veins and inferior cava vein. This is the cause of varicose veins in the lower limbs, vulva, and abdominal wall and hemorrhoids.

RESPIRATORY SYSTEM

After the 20th week, alveolar ventilation increases due to a rise in the tidal volume (TV) (i.e., an increase in the volume per minute—a change in the volume and not in the frequency). Due to diaphragm elevation, total lung capacity (TLC) is decreased by a decrease in residual volume (RV), expiratory reserve volume (ERV), and inspiratory reserve volume (IRV). This reduction in TLC is compensated for by the increase in TV; therefore, vital capacity (VC) is maintained under normal limits.

RENAL SYSTEM

During pregnancy, the kidneys increase in size and the ureters dilate due to muscular relaxation (progesterone effect) and mechanical compression on the right side and the colon sigmoids on the left side. A stasis of urine flow occurs that predispose to pyelonephritis. The glomerular filtration rate (GFR) increases 50% during the second half of pregnancy. As a result, blood urea nitrogen (BUN) and creatinine levels decrease approximately 25%. There is also an activation of the renin-angiotensin system that leads to an increase in aldosterone levels. This increase causes sodium and water retention, a physiologic event that compensates for the sodium loss due to the increase in the GFR.

GASTROINTESTINAL SYSTEM

Progesterone causes relaxation of the smooth muscle in the gastrointestinal (GI) tract. This is the cause of many of the symptoms that accompany pregnancy, such as morning sickness (due to estrogen, progesterone, and human chorionic gonadotropin [hCG] elevation), epigastric pain (lower sphincter relaxation), and constipation (due to GI stasis). There is also increased tone of the gallbladder due to stasis of the bile fluid.

ENDOCRINE

The suprarenals, thyroid gland, and hypophysis increase in size. The luteal body in the ovary produces progesterone and estrogen until the 12th week of gestation. After the 12th week, progesterone and estrogen are produced by the placenta.

Local Changes

OVARIES AND FALLOPIAN TUBES

These organs suffer hypertrophy and increase their vascularization. After the 12th week of pregnancy, the luteal body in one of the ovaries undergoes an involution and transforms itself to an albican body.

UTERINE MODIFICATIONS

In general this organ undergoes an incredible transformation, weighing about 100 g at the beginning of pregnancy and 1000 g at the end of the pregnancy. Its shape changes initially from pyriform to spheric. The vascularization and cervix change in a parallel form during the sixth to eighth weeks of pregnancy.

VAGINAL CHANGES

The changes are principally due to the increase in vascularization.

OBSTETRICS TERMINOLOGY AND DEFINITIONS

Ob/Gyn physicians use their own particular medical terms that relate to other symptoms or past events. These terms are helpful when composing a written note. Being familiar with these terms saves time and makes it easy for other health-care providers to understand the patient's problem.

Information About the Pregnancy

The following terms appear to be similar, and their meanings frequently overlap.

GRAVITY

Gravity refers to the number of times that a woman has been pregnant. A woman can be described as:

Nulligravida—never been pregnant
Primigravida—pregnant for the first time
Multigravida—has had more than one pregnancy

PARITY

Parity refers to the number of pregnancies that led to the delivery (vaginal or cesarean) of one or more products (alive or dead) with a weight of 500 g or more or that was delivered at or after 20 weeks of pregnancy. A multiple pregnancy is considered as a single parity. Parity is also subclassified as:

Nullipara. A woman who has never completed a pregnancy to the viable stage. She may or may not have aborted previously.
Primipara. A woman who has delivered one fetus or fetuses (*multiple gestation*) or who has reached the stage of viability in the current pregnancy.
Multipara. A woman who has completed two or more pregnancies to the viable stage (the number of pregnancies reaching viability does not necessarily equal the number of fetuses delivered).

Parity is further subdivided according to TPAL—**t**erm and **p**reterm deliveries, number of **a**bortions, and number of **l**iving children. These terms are described further in the following section.

4-Digit Code Obstetric Formula *(G:TPAL)*

This is a simplified form to describe the above definitions. Being familiar with this formula will allow you to save time and direct your questions more appropriately. The formula is as follows:

G:x   P: t-p-a-l

Gravity: **x** = Total number of pregnancies, including abortuses, hydatidiform moles, and ectopic pregnancies

Parity: **t** = Total number of newborns at **t**erm

p = Total number of newborns at preterm

a = Total number of abortuses (spontaneous abortion, induced abortion, and ectopic pregnancies)

l = Total number of living children

The following are examples showing the use of the obstetric formula:

Examples of Using the G:TPAL Formula

A woman who is in her third pregnancy and has two living children who were born at term would be **G3: P 2-0-0-2**

A woman who has given birth to one set of preterm twins, one term infant, and had two miscarriages would be **G4: P 1-1-2-3**

A woman who has given birth to two term infants, one premature child, one miscarriage and has been treated once with curettage due to hydatidiform mole and is currently pregnant would be **G6: P 2-1-2-3.**

DATING PREGNANCY

According to the World Health Organization (WHO), gestational age (GA) is defined by the age of the fetus in days or weeks and is measured from the last menstrual period (LMP). The developmental age (DA) is the number of days or weeks since fertilization has occurred. Because fertilization usually occurs 2 weeks after the menstrual period, the GA is 2 weeks more than the DA. The easiest method of determining the GA is with a pregnancy calendar or calculator. However, you will not be allowed to use a pregnancy calendar or calculator for the CSA exam. The GA can be calculated by three methods: knowing the date of the LMP, knowing the uterine size, and ultrasound.

Knowing the Date of the LMP

Step 1: Add 10 days to the LMP date.

Step 2: From that date, count the number of months up to the current date (today's date).

Step 3: Add 1 week for every 2 months up to the current date. For example:

LMP: 7/12/01

Step 1: LMP date plus 10 days: 7/22/01

Today's date: 12/25/01

Step 2: There have been 5 months (20 weeks) from 7/22/01 until 12/25/01

Step 3: Adding 1 week for every 2 months that have passed between 7/22/01 and 12/25/01 equals 2 additional weeks.

Gestational age: 20 weeks (step 2) + 2 weeks (step 3) = 22 weeks

Knowing the Uterine Size

This is a trusted method that helps evaluate intrauterine growth, particularly its retardation. Between 18 and 30 weeks of pregnancy, there is an excellent correlation between the size of the uterus and the GA in weeks. The measurement in centimeters from the symphysis pubis to the top of the fundus should approximate the weeks of gestation. Before 12 weeks gestation, the uterus is usually a pelvic organ (i.e., it cannot be palpated). At 12 weeks gestation, the uterus is at the level of symphysis pubis. At 20 weeks of gestation, the fundus of the uterus will be at the level of the belly button. Mc-Donald techniques are helpful to calculate the GA as follows:

$$\textbf{Uterine size (cm)} \times \textbf{8/7} = \textbf{GA in weeks}$$
$$\textbf{Uterine size (cm)} \times \textbf{2/7} = \textbf{GA in months}$$

Ultrasound

The size of the gestational sac as visualized on ultrasound can accurately predict the due date ±3 days. It is very helpful in women who have an uncertain LMP, who conceived while still breast-feeding, who recently stopped using oral contraceptives, or who have irregular menses. It is the most accurate method to estimate gestational age. It must be performed on all pregnant women between 18 and 20 weeks.

EXPECTED DATE OF CONFINEMENT (EDC)

This is calculated by using either of the following rules:

1. **Naegele rule.** This method is the one most commonly used in the United States. EDC is calculated by adding 9 months plus 7 days to the LMP date. For example, if the LMP was on 4/15/01, then the EDC will be 1/22/02. This calculation is unreliable in women with irregular menstrual cycles and in women who have been using birth control pills.
2. **Wahl rule.** This rule adds 10 days to the LMP and subtracts 3 months. In this case if the LMP was on 4/15/01, then the EDC will be 1/25/02.

Information About the Product

It is important to know the different meanings of the word *product*. Figure 4–1 provides a more descriptive orientation regarding time and terminology. The following describes terminology used about and related to the product.

Embryo. Describes the product from the time of fertilization to 8 weeks GA (10 weeks of gestation).

Fetus. The product from 8 weeks GA to the time of birth.

Newborn. The product from delivery until 28 days of age.

Infant. A child between the time of delivery up to 1 year of age.

Abortion. The termination of pregnancy before the viability of the product, approximately before the 20th week of pregnancy or if the product weighs 500 g or less. Abortion can be spontaneous (inevitable, incomplete, missed, or habitual) or induced (medical or mechanical).

Previable. A product delivered before 24 weeks of gestation.

Preterm. When a product is delivered between 24 and 37 weeks of gestation. **Premature** is the term used to describe a lack of development manifested by low birth weight (500 to 2499 g), physical signs of immaturity, and gestational age younger than 37 weeks.

Postterm. This is also called **postmaturity** or **postdatism.** It is the term that most commonly describes a dysmaturity syndrome in a pregnancy that is carried after 42 weeks. The significance of postterm pregnancy involves a significant risk to the fetus and occurs in 10% of pregnancies.

Information About the Fetus

Leopold maneuvers provide information about the presentation and position of the fetus and must be confirmed during the pelvic examination on the day of delivery. The following definitions are obtained during the physical exam by using the Leopold maneuvers. A detailed description in your written notes is mandatory if you have a pregnant SP.

FETAL HABITUS

This term indicates the relation between the different parts of the fetus (head, trunk, and limbs). This term can explain how the fetus is positioned inside of the uterine cavity. The normal habitus of the fetus is in flexion position. The fetus has an ovoid shape and has two poles (cephalic and breech pole), dorsal and ventral side. The big parts are the names used to describe the cephalic and breech poles, and the small parts are used to name the limbs.

LIE OF THE FETUS

Also termed **situation,** this is the relationship of the long axis of the fetus to the long axis of the mother. The lie can be:

Longitudinal. The fetal head is either up or down. Occurs in 99.5% of cases.

Transverse. Occurs in approximately 0.25% of cases. In this case, the fetus is crosswise in the uterine cavity.

Oblique. Occurs in approximately 0.25% of cases. This term indicates an unstable situation that can be either longitudinal or transverse during the course of labor.

(Note: In the case of transverse or oblique lie, the fetus' head indicates in which maternal side [left or right] it is.)

POSITION

This is the relationship between one part of the fetus and one of the maternal sides. If the fetus is lying in a longitudinal position, the back of the fetus determines the position depending on what side it is on. In this case, two positions can exist:

Left position. Occurs in 66% of cases.

Right position. Occurs in 34% of cases.

PRESENTATION

Fetal presentation is determined by the portion of the fetus that can be felt through the cervix, depending on how the fetus is lying.

If the fetus is longitudinal, two forms of presentation can exist:

Cephalic presentation. Occurs in 96% of cases and is subclassified as vertex (95%), face (5%), and brow (5%).

Breech presentation. Occurs in 3.5% of cases and is subclassified as frank, complete, and footling.

If the fetal lie is transverse or oblique, the presented part is the shoulder. This occurs in 0.5% of cases.

FETAL WEIGHT (FW)

Intrauterine fetal weight can be calculated by knowing the uterine size (US) in centimeters and using the Johnson method. This method is important to use when the physician must decide whether to proceed with the pregnancy until labor occurs, to induce labor, to use tocolytics agents, or to perform a cesarean section (C-section). This method is useful only if the presentation of the fetus is cephalic.

$$FW = (US - n) \times 155 \pm 100 \text{ g, where}$$

n can take two values:

$$n = 11 \text{ if engagement has occurred}$$

$$n = 12 \text{ if engagement has not occurred}$$

You are not expected to estimate this value during the CSA exam, but you can do it and include it in your notes if you are good at mathematics!

Information About Uterine Bleeding

Be familiar with the following terms, because you will need to use them correctly in your written notes.

Dysfunctional uterine bleeding (DUB). This is excessive uterine bleeding with no demonstrable organic cause. It is often associated with anovulation due to an endocrine problem. DUB is a diagnosis of exclusion.

Intermenstrual bleeding. Intermenstrual bleeding is variable bleeding that occurs between regular menstrual periods.

Dysmenorrhea. Dysmenorrhea describes chronic, cyclic pelvic pain that accompanies menstruation. It can be primary (no clinically identifiable cause) or secondary (occurs in the presence of organic, identifiable disease).

Mittelschmerz. This is chronic, cyclic pelvic pain that is sudden, episodic, and unilateral in the lower abdomen. It can be caused by minor bleeding from rupture of the follicle into the abdominal cavity.

Menorrhagia (hypermenorrhea). This describes prolonged (more than 7 days) and excessive (80 mL or greater) uterine bleeding that occurs at regular intervals. (The average blood loss in a normal menses is approximately 35 mL.) Patients describe the bleeding as pouring or gushing and use more than 24 pads a day (soaking more than 1 pad/hour). It can be caused by fibroids, endometrial hyperplasia, adenomyosis, polyps, endometrial or cervical cancer, DUB, bleeding disorders, or pregnancy complications.

Metrorrhagia. In metrorrhagia, bleeding is usually the same as in regular menses but occurs at irregular intervals. It can be caused by fibroids, endometrial hyperplasia, adenomyosis, polyps, endometrial or cervical cancer, and pregnancy complications.

Polymenorrhea. Polymenorrhea is a uterine bleeding disorder that occurs at regular intervals less than 21 days from each other. The bleeding episodes are similar. It is usually caused by anovulation. Polymenorrhea is sometimes mistakenly diagnosed as metrorrhagia.

Oligomenorrhea. This is an infrequent uterine bleeding disorder that occurs in intervals more than 35 days from each other. It reflects a disruption of the pituitary-gonadal axis by hypothalamic, pituitary, or gonadal abnormalities or systemic diseases. The most common cause is pregnancy.

Hypomenorrhea. In hypomenorrhea, the flow of menses is usually light. It is usually seen in patients with hypogonadotropic hypogonadism, in athletes, and in patients with anorexia. It is also seen in atrophic endometrium, Asherman syndrome, and in patients using oral contraceptives or Depo-Provera (medroxyprogesterone). Other causes include cervical stenosis or congenital anomalies.

Lochia. Lochia is uterine discharge that follows delivery and lasts for 3 to 4 weeks. It can appear in three forms:

Lochia rubra. Appears during the first few days after delivery. It has a bloody content and it stains.

Lochia serosa. Appears on the 3rd to 4th day after delivery, is paler than lochia rubra, and has a mixed content of blood and serum.

Lochia alba. Appears after the 10th day, because of the mixture of leukocytes, and is yellowish.

Watery vaginal secretion in late pregnancy. This is a sign of possible rupture of membranes (ROM) in pregnancy. If it occurs before 37 weeks GA, it is considered preterm ROM. If it occurs before the onset of labor, it is called premature ROM. The ROM normally precedes delivery, which should occur in the following 24 hours. If ROM occurs and labor does not begin, this should raise the suspicion of chorioamnionitis. Table 4–1 lists a differential diagnosis of this symptom. Table 4–2 presents a differential diagnosis of uterine bleeding.

TABLE 4–1. Watery Vaginal Secretion in Late Pregnancy

Differential Diagnosis	Diagnostic Workup
1. Rupture of membranes (ROM) (preterm or premature)	1. Pelvic/speculum examination
2. Vaginosis (bacterial, yeast, or protozoan)	2. Nitrazine and fern tests
3. Urinary tract infection (UTI)	3. Urinalysis
	4. Wet prep of vaginal swab
	5. Whiff test
	6. Group B streptococci culture

PRESUMPTIVE SIGNS AND SYMPTOMS OF PREGNANCY

There are signs and symptoms related to the general modifications of pregnancy that are not diagnostic, because other physiologic and pathologic states can cause the same changes. The following signs and symptoms are positive when evaluating a possible pregnancy.

Amenorrhea. The patient's period should be at least 10 days late before this is considered as a reliable indication of pregnancy.

Breast changes. This is a relatively reliable sign in early pregnancy. Complaints are usually of tenderness (mastodynia) and tingling. Breast enlargement is evident during the second month. Calostrum secretion may begin after the 16th week of pregnancy.

Skin changes. See Physiology of Pregnancy section, General Changes.

Nausea and vomiting. Nausea can occur with or without vomiting, usually begins during the 4th to 6th weeks of gestation, and does not last longer than the first trimester. It has a morning presentation.

Urinary disturbances. In early pregnancy, the growing uterus creates pressure over the bladder. This symptom usually resolves when the uterus continues to grow outside the pelvic cavity. However, it returns in late pregnancy because of the pressure exerted by the fetal head.

Basal temperature. There is an increase in the basal temperature of 0.3°C to 0.6°C.

Fatigue. General fatigue, vertigo, and headaches are common.

Fetal movement. Known as quickening, this is frequently described as gas bubbles and appears during the 16th to 20th weeks of gestation.

TABLE 4–2. Abnormal Uterine Bleeding

Differential Diagnosis	Diagnostic Workup
1. Endometrial hyperplasia	1. Pelvic/speculum examination
2. Endometrial polyps	2. Pap smear
3. Endometrial cancer	3. Endometrial biopsy
4. Cervical cancer	4. Pregnancy test/quantitative beta-human chorionic gonadotropin (hCG)
5. Trophoblastic disease	
6. Pregnancy complication	5. Pelvic ultrasound
7. Ectopic pregnancy	6. Diagnostic dilation and curettage
8. Dysfunctional uterine bleeding	

Signs and Symptoms of Probable Pregnancy

These signs and symptoms constitute clinical evidence of pregnancy. They are not exclusive to pregnancy, but their presence provides a strong suspicion.

Amenorrhea. See previous definition.

Enlargement of the abdomen. After the 12th week of pregnancy, the uterus can be palpated through the abdominal wall as a small medial mass at the level of the symphysis pubis. At the 20th week the uterus will be at the level of the umbilicus or belly button.

Uterine changes. As the uterus enlarges it suffers some anatomic changes that can be noted on a complete gynecologic examination (bimanual and speculum examination). You are not expected to perform a vaginal examination during the CSA exam.

Ballottement of the uterus. During the 16th to 20th weeks of pregnancy, a floating object is perceived as occupying the uterine cavity.

Uterine souffle. This is a whisper or rush sound found on auscultation that is synchronous with the pulse of the mother.

Definitive Signs of Pregnancy

The following factors determine the definitive diagnosis of pregnancy.

FETAL HEART BEAT (FHR) IDENTIFICATION

This is performed by one of the following methods:

Auscultation. By using a stethoscope, fetoscope, or Pinnar bell, the FHR can be heard between 17 and 19 weeks of gestation.

Ultrasound. FHR can be identified between 12 and 14 weeks of gestation by ultrasound fetal heart monitor.

SONOGRAPHIC VISUALIZATION OF THE FETUS

This can be used to identify the gestational ring, embryo, and fetal heart motion. The time to identify those structures varies depending on the type of ultrasound probe (vaginal or abdominal). By using abdominal ultrasound, a gestational sac is initially seen at 5 to 6 weeks of pregnancy. Vaginal ultrasound can detect a pregnancy at 3 to 4 weeks.

Prenatal Care

The main objective of prenatal care is the delivery of a healthy infant and maintenance of the health of the mother. One of the goals is to identify a high-risk patient at an early stage and begin appropriate treatment as soon as possible. Prenatal care has the following characteristics.

IT MUST BE STARTED IMMEDIATELY

Pregnancy should be suspected in any sexually active woman as soon as she detects the absence of menses. Prenatal care must be initiated immediately after a diagnosis has been made (i.e., pregnancy has been confirmed).

IT MUST BE PERIODIC

Prenatal care must be periodic and repetitive, beginning with a comprehensive history and physical exam to identify risk factors or abnormalities. Care should continue at regular intervals as follows:

1. From 1 to 30 weeks GA (until the 6th month). Prenatal visits once a month.
2. From 31 to 35 weeks GA (during the 7th month). Prenatal visits every 15 days.
3. After 36 weeks GA until delivery. Prenatal visits every week.

IT MUST BE COMPLETE

Prenatal care must consist of a general evaluation and be focused on the present pregnancy. Special emphasis should be placed on the obstetric history of prior pregnancies, including dates, outcomes, modes of delivery, amount of time spent in labor, birth weight, and puerperium.

INITIAL VISIT

The physician needs to take a medical history, perform a physical exam, and prescribe a battery of initial laboratory tests (Table 4–3). The major goals are to confirm the pregnancy, evaluate the GA, detect any obstetric risks, start an appropriate plan for follow-up visits, and reference the appropriate level of attention the patient requires.

ROUTINE VISITS

The schedule of follow-up visits will be explained to the patient during the initial visit. Follow-up prenatal care visits are routine events.

At every visit, pay special attention to the following:

Danger signals. Any vaginal bleeding, swelling of the face or fingers, headaches, blurred vision, or abdominal pain are danger signals. You must make the patient aware of the need to contact you (or the treating physician) as soon as possible if any of these signs occur (Table 4–4).

Maternal weight. The American College of Obstetricians and Gynecologists recommend a weight gain of 10 to 12 kg (22 to 27 lb) for the average pregnancy. Underweight women may have to gain more, whereas obese women should gain only 6

TABLE 4–3. Laboratory Tests Performed in Pregnancy

First Trimester (Initial Visit)	Second Trimester	Third Trimester
Hemoglobin and hematocrit	MSAFP (between 16 and 18 weeks)	1-hr glucose tolerance test
Blood group and Rh factor	Ultrasound (between 18 and 20 weeks)	Repeat gonorrhea and chlamydia**
Glucose levels*	Amniocentesis//	Group B streptococci
RPR screen		Chest radiograph††
Rubella antibody screen		
HIV test†		
Hepatitis B		
Surface antigen		
Chlamydia culture		
PPD		
Gonorrhea culture		
Pap smear		
Urinalysis		
Urine culture		
Sickle cell test‡		
Toxoplasma titers§		

MSAFP = maternal serum alpha-fetoprotein; PPD = purified protein derivative; RPR = rapid plasma reagin.
*Indicated in patients with a family history of diabetes, previous large infants, and glucosuria.
†Should be offered but is not performed routinely.
‡Tests for sickle cell anemia in black patients with positive family histories. Sickle trait is not a risk.
§Should be performed on any women with cat(s) in her home.
//Should be performed in patients of advanced maternal age (older than 35 years)
**Should be performed in high-risk patients.
††Should be performed if purified protein derivative (PPD) is positive.
(Adapted with permission from Callahan T, Caughey A, Heffner L: *Blueprints in Obstetrics and Gynecology.* Boston: Blackwell Science Inc., 1998, p 5.)

TABLE 4–4. Signs of Labor

True Labor	False Labor	Warning Signs*
Contractions at regular intervals that regularly shorten	Contractions that occur at irregular intervals	Any watery vaginal secretion
		Vaginal bleeding
The intensity of contractions increases progressively, more that 1 minute	Contraction intervals are long and do not establish any regular pattern. Intensity is the same	Severe headaches
		Blurred vision, tinnitus
		Painful cramps in abdomen and back
Discomfort in the back and abdomen	Discomfort is chiefly in the lower abdomen	Intense nausea and vomiting
Progressive dilation of the cervix	Contractions do not cause cervical dilation	Syncope, vertigo, sudden increase in weight, oliguria
		Edema of face and limbs
Contractions are not affected by sedation	Contractions are usually stopped by sedation	Loss of fetal movements

*The patient must to be instructed to look for these signs and to contact her treating physician when they occur.
(Adapted with permission from Beck WW: *NMS Obstetrics and Gynecology,* 2e. Philadelphia: Lippincott Williams and Wilkins, 1989, p 32.)

to 9 kg (15 to 20 lb). As described previously, during the first trimester maternal weight tends to remain the same or decreases due to vomiting. During the second trimester, weight gain can be 1200 g/month. During the third trimester, the increase in weight tends to be 1500 g/month but is less during the lasts 2 weeks. The weight increase during the third trimester should not be more than 500 g/week. Any increase greater than this should raise the suspicion of fluid retention (preeclampsia).

Control of vital signs. Vital signs should be monitored, especially blood pressure.

Measurement of fundal height. If the fundal height is progressively decreasing or 3 cm less than GA, an ultrasound evaluation must be ordered.

Examination of legs. Special attention should be paid to edemas, varicose veins, and tendinous hyperreflexia.

Laboratory assessment. Review any laboratory results.

At every visit from 26 weeks GA on, pay attention to all factors mentioned above plus the following:

Fetal examination. Fetal lie, position, and presentation.

Assessment of fetal movement. Ten movements per day is considered normal.

Assessment of fetal heart rate. Normal fetal heart rate is 120 to 160 bpm.

Laboratory tests. As clinical criteria dictate (see Table 4–3).

At every visit from 36 weeks GA on, pay attention to all factors mentioned above plus the following:

Fetopelvic examination in primigravidas. This can be performed by measuring the pelvic diameters manually. On the CSA exam, limit this to ordering it on the diagnostic workup plan in the written notes. You are not expected to do this on the exam day.

Determine fetal engagement. This is the mechanism by which the biparietal diameter of the head passes through the pelvic inlet.

Reevaluation of the general maternal state.

Laboratory tests. As clinical criteria dictate (see Table 4–3).

OBSTETRICS AND GYNECOLOGY WRITTEN NOTES

Ob/Gyn notes are similar to general medical written notes in many aspects. The major difference in Ob/Gyn notes is that they are mostly focused on descriptions related to the female reproductive system (gynecology). The major task in taking an obstetrics history is identifying a high-risk patient. Information about socioeconomic status, the age of the woman, and drug abuse need to be taken into consideration. Continuous assessment as described in the Prenatal Care section is imperative. The history and clinical exam will vary depending on the stage of the pregnancy and the patient's symptoms.

Figure 4–2 is a common guideline for the clinical Ob/Gyn history.

Patients Who Have Been Raped

One important aspect that must be considered is the presentation of a patient who has been raped. Rape is considered a violent crime in the United States, but its definition varies depending on the legislation of the individual state. Legal codes may categorize rape depending on the anatomic site of the assault (oral, anal, or vaginal) and the degree of penetration that has occurred (none, slight, or full). History taking about the sexual assault is uncomfortable for victims and the examiner, but it should not cause additional trauma. Always try to create a safe and secure environment. The psychologic effect is not related to the degree of penetration, and some victims of sexual assault characteristically perceive themselves as guilty of causing the assault, especially in situations in which they used poor judgment (hitch-hiking). The physical exam must be performed in a nonjudgmental way. Sexual assault victims should undergo a complete general physical examination, including a pelvic exam. The medical history must contain detailed information about the assault: grade of penetration, ejaculation (yes or no), location of ejaculation, was the victim drunk, if the victim has bathed. Also document if the patient has douched, voided, or defecated. This information is important because these factors can alter sample results.

Remember to prescribe antibiotic prophylaxis to all adult victims. Recommended regimens include doxycycline 100 mg by mouth twice a day for 7 days, and ceftriaxone (250 mg intramuscularly once). Table 4–5 lists the differential diagnosis and steps that need to be considered when treating rape victims.

Patients Who Have Suffered Domestic Abuse

During their lifetimes, 25% to 50% of women experience domestic violence. One in five women who presents to the emergency department has been injured by her partner. Domestic violence is usually cyclic and repetitive; in 90% of cases, there is a history of police intervention. Victims of domestic violence frequently seek consultation due to

---

A) OBSTETRIC/GYNECOLOGIC HISTORY
1. Chief complaint (CC)
2. History of the present illness (HPI)
3. Present pregnancy (PP)
4. Obstetric and gynecologic history (Ob/GynH)
5. Past medical history (PMH)
6. Social history (SH)
7. Family history (FH)

B) PHYSICAL EXAMINATION
1. General examination (GE)
2. HEENT
3. Neck
4. Chest ---► *Breasts*
          ---► *Respiratory system*
          ---► *Heart*
5. Abdomen
6. Obstetric and gynecologic examination
7. Extremities ---► check edema
8. Neuro ---► check hyperreflexia

C) DIFFERENTIAL DIAGNOSIS
–Plans for dif. diagnosis (1-5)

D) DIAGNOSTIC WORKUP
–Plans for diagnosis (1-5)
–Plans for rectal/pelvic/female breast

FIGURE 4–2. The obstetrics and gynecology format of a patient note. Indicate on the diagnostic workup but do not perform either a breast, rectal, or pelvic exam. HEENT = head, ears, eyes, nose, throat.

TABLE 4-5. Treating Rape Victims

Differential Diagnosis	Diagnostic Workup
1. Sexual assault	1. Genital/pelvic examination
2. Domestic violence	2. UV or Wood light to observe dry fluorescent seminal fluid
3. Posttraumatic stress disorder	
4. Dissociative disorder	3. Saline samples from mouth, anus, and cervical pool
	4. Comb the pubic hair and store the sample in a plastic bag and label it
	5. Pap smear
	6. Laboratory tests: Veneral Disease Research Laboratory (VDRL), blood type, beta-human chorionic gonadotropin (hCG), human immunodeficiency virus (HIV), hepatitis B

chronic pelvic pain, sexual dysfunctions, low interest in sex, arousal problems, dyspareunia, and anxiety. You can assess the patient by asking the following questions:

How are you and your partner getting along?
What happens when you disagree with your partner?
How do you resolve any conflict between you and your partner?
Have you ever been physically abused, pressured, or forced into a sexual or nonsexual situation?

The differential diagnosis and workup plan for these patients are shown in Table 4–6.

Adolescent Patients

Be prepared for attending to an adolescent patient who comes to you requesting oral contraceptives. This situation must be considered as any other physician-patient interaction. If the patient is competent and aware, explain the benefits and risks of contraception and reassure her that the information exchanged will not be released to anyone, including her parents. Figure 4–2 is the format of the parameters of an obstetric and gynecology medical note for the CSA exam.

OBSTETRICS AND GYNECOLOGY MEDICAL HISTORY

Chief Complaint

Focus on the patient's age, history of major illnesses, and the immediate problem. Age is a very important factor that you must mention in your notes. Review Table 4–7, which shows the risk factors related to maternal age. Begin the discussion by asking the patient, *How can I help you?* or *What kind of problem do you have?*

TABLE 4-6. Treating Victims of Domestic Violence

Differential Diagnosis	Diagnostic Workup
1. Domestic violence	1. Discussion with the domestic violence support system
2. Somatoform disorders	2. Photographic documentation of any bruises or lesions
3. Posttraumatic stress disorder	3. Radiographs if obvious lesions exist
4. Dissociative disorder	4. Patient follow-up
5. Sexual assault	5. Psychiatric assessment

TABLE 4–7. Pregnancy Risk Factors Related to Maternal Age

Younger than 20 Years of Age	Older than 35 Years of Age
Premature births	First trimester miscarriages
Fetal deaths	Genetically abnormal conceptuses (trisomy
Preeclampsia and eclampsia	21-neonatal deaths 90%–, trisomies 13 and 18)
Uterine dysfunction	Preeclampsia and eclampsia
Late maternal care	Maternal and fetal death
	Diabetes, hypertension
	Multiple gestations
	Labor problems

(Adapted with permission from Beck WW: *NMS Obstetrics and Gynecology,* 2e. Philadelphia: Lippincott Williams and Wilkins, 1989, p 76.)

See the following examples of writing notes about the chief complaint:

Chief Compliant (Ob)

Kathy is a 22 yo pregnant woman who presents with abdominal pain, stating that she was leaking fluid from the vagina.

Chief C. (Ob)

Ms. Collins is a 29-year-old w. woman in her third trimester of pregnancy, stating that she had painless vaginal bleeding.

C. Compliant (Gyn)

Temika is a 42-year-old b. female who states that she is having hot flushing, perspiration, and insomnia.

CC (Gyn)

Ms. Garland is a 19-year-old w. female, previously well, who came to the emergency room with abdominal pain, chills, and vaginal bleeding.

History of the Present Illness

Describe exactly the patient's problem and symptoms. Mention location, duration, etc. Many of the symptoms that you will encounter on the CSA exam will be common complaints, such as symptoms related to urinary tract infections (UTIs), vaginal bleeding problems, incontinence, and endocrine problems. To include all of the above complaints is beyond the scope of this book. Some tables in this chapter deal with particular aspects commonly seen by the general physician. Table 4–8 shows some complications commonly seen during pregnancy. Vaginal bleeding is a common complaint during pregnancy. In the United States, hemorrhage is the leading cause of maternal death. The possible cause of bleeding varies depending of the stage of pregnancy. Table 4–9 lists a differential diagnosis of bleeding in pregnancy.

See the following examples or review general written medical notes in Chapter 3.

History of the Present Illness (Ob)

This pregnant woman reported having an increase in the intensity and frequency of colic type pain. At the moment it is mostly in the lower abdomen and in the back. She also reported that she had been leaking a clear white fluid an hour before coming here.

TABLE 4-8. Common Complications of Pregnancy

First Trimester	Second Trimester	Third Trimester
Bleeding (25% of all pregnancies bleed; half of these end in abortion) Hyperemesis gravidarum	Incompetent cervix Premature ROM, preterm labor Bleeding (due to low-lying placenta)	Premature ROM Bleeding (due to a normal stretching of cervix, placenta previa, abruptio placentae)

ROM = rupture of membranes.

HPI (Ob)

Patient states that she was well until two weeks ago, when she noted difficulty in wearing her tennis shoes. She had no other symptoms until yesterday, when she developed frontal headache and epigastric pain. She denies visual disturbances or seizures.

H. of the Present Illness (Ob/Gyn)

The patient has been treated with ampicillin 500 mg qid 7/10 due to a urinary tract infection, but was well until today when she developed chills, dysuria, urgency, and left flank pain.

HPI (Gyn)

The patient reported having been treated with danazol for endometriosis four months ago. She was fine until 2 week ago when she noticed weight gain, decrease in breast size, dyspareunia and oily skin.

TABLE 4-9. Bleeding Causes During Pregnancy

First Trimester	Second Trimester	Third Trimester	Postpartum
Differential Diagnosis			
1. Intrauterine abortion (threatened, incomplete, and complete)	1. Abortions (threatened, incomplete, and complete)	1. Placenta previa	1. Uterine atony
		2. Abruptio placentae	2. Retained products of conception (POCs)
2. Ectopic pregnancy	2. Postcoital bleeding	3. Fetal vessel rupture	3. Placenta accreta
3. Molar pregnancy	3. Cervical vaginal lesions	4. Bleeding due to normal stretching cervix	4. Vaginal cervical laceration
4. Postcoital bleeding	4. Premature labor	5. Uterine rupture‡	
	5. Bleeding due to low-lying placenta		
Diagnostic Workup			
1. Pelvic examination	1. Pelvic examination	1. Pelvic ultrasound	1. Pelvic/speculum examination
2. Pelvic ultrasound	2. Pelvic ultrasound	2. CBC	
3. CBC	3. CBC	3. Electronic fetal monitoring	2. CBC
4. Serial beta-hCG*	4. Serial beta-hCG	4. Pelvic exam§	3. Pelvic ultrasound
5. Blood type†	5. Blood type		4. PT, PTT

CBC = complete blood count; beta-hCG = beta-human chorionic gonadotropin; PT = prothrombin time; PTT = partial thromboplastin time.

*Quantitative: In normal uterine pregnancy the trophoblastic tissue secretes beta-hCG, which doubles every 48 hours.

†If the patient knows that she is Rh-negative, request the Kleihauer-Betke test to estimate the correct dose of RhoGAM.

‡May occur during labor, associated with oxytocin overuse. Shock, hypovolemic symptoms, and pain are present.

§Depends on the etiology. Contraindicated in placenta previa. This maneuver can be performed in the operating room.

Present Pregnancy

You can skip this section if the SP is not pregnant. Obtain information about the current pregnancy and the patient's general status (appetite, thirst, urination, mood, and sleep). The information that you need to obtain is as follows:

1. Last menstrual period (LMP)
2. Expected date of confinement (EDC)
3. Gestational age (GA)
4. 4-Digit code obstetric formula (G:TPAL)

Review the following written medical notes about the present pregnancy; assume that the current calculation dates for the first and second examples are 12/20/01 and 11/12/01, respectively.

Present Pregnancy

Patient states that she is asymptomatic, no major complaints

Last menstrual period: 9/02/01

Expected date of confinement: 6/9/02

Gestational age: 13 weeks

Obstetric formula: G2: P-1-0-0-1

P. Pregnancy

The patient reports low back pain, normal appetite and normal sleeping hours. No mood alterations. LMP was 03/14/01; EDC: 12/21/01; GA: 36 weeks; Gravity 2, Parity-0-0-1-0.

Ob/Gyn History

This is a very important part of the clinical history. You must be explicit, but in a simple manner for CSA purposes. This reflects the patient's gynecologic functional history and problems as well as the history of normal or abnormal pregnancies. The information that you need to obtain is as follows:

1. Age at menarche
2. Last menstrual period (LMP) (referring to the LMP of any child-bearing, pregnant, or nonpregnant woman)
3. Age at menopause
4. Last Pap smear
5. Birth control method(s)
6. Characteristics of menses
7. HIV risk factors
8. Other
9. Previous pregnancies

Use your own criteria for a particular question, depending on the case presented to you. Age at menarche, LMP, age at menopause, and birth control method(s) are self-explanatory. Under last Pap smear, report the date and the result if the SP can provide it. For characteristics of menses focus on the regularity, frequency, and duration of periods (e.g., 4/28 means 4 days duration every 28 days); the amount of bleeding; bleeding between periods; and bleeding after intercourse. You can count the number of pads used per day by asking the patient the number of pads soaked. For more information see the Information About Uterine Bleeding section in this chapter. Regarding menopause, obtain information about menopausal symptoms, postmenopausal bleeding, estrogen therapy, and age of presentation if pertinent. Screen for possible HIV risk factors, such as transfusions, intravenous (IV) drug use, and multiple sexual partners. Other information can be about the patient's sexual relationship(s), libido, sexual difficulties, and abnormalities (such as vaginal discharge, vulvar itching, and venereal diseases and their treatments). For previous pregnancies focus on miscarriages, surgical procedures, or other complications. Concentrate on the length of gestation, length of labor, fetal presentation, type of delivery (premature, preterm, term), birth, birth weight, and fetal outcome. Some patients may have had several miscarriages. The definition of a patient who has had recurrent abortions is someone with three or more consecutives spontaneous abortions. This problem is discussed in Table 4–10.

See the following examples of Ob/Gyn history medical notes:

OB & Gyn History (Ob)

Menarche at 13 yo, LMP on July 12, 1998, Pap smear 6 months ago, result: normal. Birth control before pregnancy with oral contraceptives, Menstruation 3/30. No previous blood transfusions, no drug use, no alterations in her sexual life.

OB&Gyn History (Gyn)

Menarche at 12 yo, LMP: 12/07/98, Pap smear never done. No birth control. Oligomenorrhea 3/43. No drug use. She's divorced with one child. She has multiple sexual partners. Positive malodorous vaginal discharge.

OB & Gyn H (Gyn)

Menarche at 12 years old, Menopause at 42 yo. Pap smear 1 year ago, result: normal. Previous gestations unremarkable.

Past Medical History

This should contain information similar to that described in Chapter 3. Divide this section into medical, surgical, and psychiatric problems, medications, etc. Direct your questions to problems that would relate to the pregnancy or to positive risk factors and to maternal mortality (hypertension, diabetes, thyroid disease, infectious diseases). For surgical questions concentrate on previous gynecologic surgeries (uterine surgeries C-sections, cervical cone biopsies). Ask about any medications that the SP has been taking. For example, exposure to Diethylstilbestrol (DES) is related to cervical incompetence and cervical adenocarcinoma. Exogenous androgens, minoxidil, phenytoin, and diazoxide may cause hirsutism. The following general parameters should be incorporated:

1. Past medical illnesses
2. Past surgical illnesses
3. Psychiatric illnesses

TABLE 4–10. **Treating Patients Who Have Had Recurrent Abortions**

Differential Diagnosis	Diagnostic Workup
1. Chromosomal abnormalities	1. Karyotype, both parents
2. Infections (rubella, toxoplasms)	2. Pelvic examination
3. Uterine anatomic defects	3. Hysterosalpingography
4. Endocrine (hypothyroidism)	4. Thyroid-stimulating hormone (TSH), thyroxine (T_4)
5. Immunologic (antiphospholipid antibody syndrome)	5. Fasting serum glucose
6. Cervical incompetence	6. Antiphospholipid antibodies
7. Maternal systemic disease (diabetes, hypertension, anemia)	7. Progesterone level on luteal phase

4. Allergies
5. Medications

For more information and examples, see Chapter 3. See the following examples of written medical notes for past medical history.

PMH

Appendectomy three years ago without complications, no medical problems were mentioned.
Medications: Iron 200 mg + folic acid 1 mg QD.
Allergies: None known.
Smoking*: 1/2 ppd since 18 years old.
EtOH*: 1 beer a day.
*Can be also mentioned in Social History

Past Med. Hist.

Patient reported having underwent right breast surgery to remove two benign cysts in 1967, hysterectomy in 1985. Back surgery for discopathy in 1991 and she is currently treated for HTN with Chlorothiazide 250 mg PO qd. She denies allergies.

Social History

This is elaborated in the same manner as in the written medical notes in Chapter 3. For example, occupation, marital status, and sexual orientation and practices are included in this section. Keep in mind that low socioeconomic status is related to an increased risk of perinatal morbidity and mortality. Socioeconomic status (SES) refers to a group of factors that play an important role in morbidity and mortality. These factors are educational level, marital status, income, and occupation. Income alone is not a determinant of high or low SES. The following are examples of social history notes.

Social History

She is married with three children, works as a cashier in a grocery store. She is sexually active and denies any other social problems.

SH

She has been unemployed for several years. She depends on food stamps for her support, and she is a single mother with three children. She is a heterosexual woman with multiple sexual partners.

Family History

Breast cancer, diabetes, and blood dyscrasias (sickle cell anemia) are important factors that should be ruled out. To complete this section of the medical note, you will depend on the circumstances described in general written medical notes (see Chapter 3).

PHYSICAL EXAMINATION

In general, this part of the medical history follows the same order as the general written medical notes in Chapter 3; there are some variations that are particular according to the age, sex, and clinical status of the patient. The same recommendations regarding written notes are given: stay calm during the CSA exam, organize your questions and ideas, and perform pertinent clinical tests as you would do with a real patient. The following are recommendations for writing an Ob/Gyn medical note.

General Examination

This is performed in the same manner as described in Chapter 3: examine the patient's external habitus, personal hygiene, facial expression, etc.

For pregnant women, describe posture, facial expression, and gait (see more information in the Physiology of Pregnancy section, General Changes). Always consider measuring height and weight. Women of short stature tend to have small babies and are at risk for low-birth-weight newborns and preterm delivery.

An inadequate progressive weight gain may reflect a nutritional deficit or maternal illness. These are associated with poor fundal growth, small fetuses, and small placentas; in simple terms, there will be fetal growth retardation. In the general document, the weight, height, and vital signs occupy one or two sentences. The following are some examples:

General Examination

Mildly ill appearing, no apparent distress observed.
T: 39.5°C, BP: 130/85 mm Hg, P: 100/min, R: 28 resp/min, Height: 1.54 m, Weight: 55 Kg

General Examination

A nervous pregnant woman, with moderate sweating.
T: 37.8°C, BP: 130/90 mmHg, P: 100/min, R: 18 resp/min, H: 1.6 m, W: 62.5 kg

General

T: 38°C, BP: 130/80, P: 74 b/min, RR: 16 r/min, H: 1.7 m, W: 60 Kg

General Exam.

At the time of presentation the patient was in moderate distress. Patient's blood pressure was 110/60 mm Hg, P: 85 b/min, R: 18 r/min, H: 1.5 m, W: 62 Kg

HEENT

HEENT refers to head, eyes, ears, nose, and throat (see Chapter 3). If you prefer, you can write your notes as Head, Eyes, and ENT. The following are examples of HEENT medical notes.

HEENT (Extended form)

Head: Normocephalic and free of visible lesions. Facial musculature revealed normal movement and adequate animation. Facial expression was consistent with an indication of the perceived pain about which the patient was complaining.

Eyes: Ocular movements were normal. Conjutivae clear without abnormalities.

Ear, nose, and throat: Pinnae were normal on inspection. Ear canals showed no evidence of scarring or deformity on inspection. Nasal septum showed no deviation. Tongue on the midline and normal movement of the soft palate were noted. There was no deficit in phonation.

HEENT *(Abbreviated form)*

Normocephalic and free of visible lesions.

Conjunctivae mildly injected with yellowish rheum bilaterally.

Ear, nose, and throat were normal.

Neck

See Chapter 3.

Chest

The cardiovascular and respiratory systems were described in Chapter 3, but some considerations are important to review. Cardiovascular diseases are the most important non-obstetric causes of disability and death in pregnant women. Ideally, a patient with known heart disease should consult her physician before becoming pregnant, but some heart diseases are manifested during pregnancy. Pre-pregnancy planning must include an exercise tolerance test. Heart disease in a pregnant woman is classified by using functional disability according to the New York Heart Association (see Chapter 3). General heart problems acquired during pregnancy are shown in Table 4–11.

According to CSA rules, you are not allowed to perform a breast exam during the CSA exam. Normally, as an examiner, if you find an abnormal mass you need to describe the characteristics, consistency, size described in centimeters, skin appearance, etc. However, during the CSA exam, you are not allowed to do this. You can ask the SP to describe the size and consistency of the apparent mass and compare it with a *pea, lemon,* or *walnut.* You can ask questions such as, *Is it as big as a lemon or a pea? Does the walnut have a shell?* The SP's answers will give you an idea of the tumor size and its consistency. In your notes or diagram, you can note it as follows: *The breast mass is described as hard as a pea and with dimples on the skin.* (Figure 4–3.)

The following paragraphs describe some important aspects of the female breast exam that you can apply during the CSA exam according to the permitted rules. Not all of the information in this section can be applied directly to the case presented to you. Use your own criteria.

FEMALE BREAST

This part of the medical exam can be difficult to perform if you do not have any experience with examining female patients. Always remember that you must be polite, courteous, and professional when you refer to or ask questions about this area. Ask the SP to be very descriptive when she refers to a problem on her breast. You do not need to perform a breast exam but you can examine her axiles to look for nodes. For descriptive purposes, the breast can be divided in four quadrants intersected perpendicular to each other at the level of the nipple, plus an extra portion that corresponds to the superior external sides of each breast corresponding to the tail of Spence. The quadrants are the upper outer, upper inner, lower outer, and lower inner, corresponding to the right or left breast, respectively (see Figure 4–3).

TABLE 4–11. Heart Problems During Pregnancy

Rheumatic heart disease

Mitral valve disease

Cardiomyopathies

Myocarditis

Aortic dissection

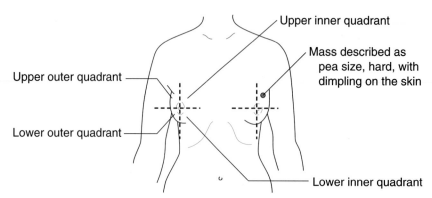

FIGURE 4–3. Diagram of a breast mass as described by the standardized patient.

Document in your notes any important signs or symptoms, such as mass localization and presence or absence of nodes, in your notes. If you consider it necessary, you can draw a breast diagram divided by the quadrants to document your findings and indicate the location of the apparent tumoral mass according to the patient's description (see Figure 4–3). The signs are more important than the symptoms in breast diseases. A review of normal physiology will help you to understand some common complaints regarding the female breast.

Thelarche is usually the first phenotypic sign of puberty. It occurs at approximately 11 years of age and is a response to an increase in estrogen. Black girls have the tendency to be more advanced in their secondary sex characteristics than white girls of the same age. Breast buds appear, and further enlargement of the breast and areolae follows. The breast undergoes cyclic changes during each menstrual cycle. In the postmenstrual phase, the pituitary gland produces follicle-stimulating hormone (FSH), which causes ovarian follicle ripening. This leads to an increase in estrogen production by the ovary, which causes proliferation of the breast ductal system. When ovulation occurs, in mid cycle, estrogen and progesterone production from the ovary decreases and the breast ducts begin to diminish. It is preferable to examine the breast gland on the days after menstruation, especially in a woman of child-bearing age, because the breasts are less sensitive and tender. During pregnancy estrogen and progesterone levels remain relatively high, causing hypertrophy and budding of the ductal system. The breasts enlarge and become darker and more erectile; colostrum can be expressed after the sixth week of gestation. At menopause there is a loss of breast parenchyma and an increase in fibrous tissue; the size diminishes and atrophy begins.

Breast pain is frequently seen in teenagers and young women, especially on the days before menstruation. This pain has a cyclic presentation and disappears at the beginning of menses. The most common complaint is breast pain radiated to the axilae. Pain that is not cyclic and is well localized can suggest the presence of a benign tumor, as in cases of fibroadenoma or localized cystic disease. Pain is not a common symptom of breast cancer, but pain that is intermittent, acute, and in a single breast can suggest a neoplasm. Any watery and bloody discharge is seen as a spot on the bra. Breast retractions can be caused by cancer and traumatic necrosis of the fatty tissue. Information about menstruation, reproduction, and hormone therapy should be recorded.

Clinical Exam

Before proceeding with the exam of the axillae, you need to explain what you are going to do, step by step. Also explain that you are only going to examine the axilae area. Explain to the SP that she must wear the gown so that the buttons/openings are in the front and that she must be seated on the side of the exam table. Stand in front of the SP and palpate the lymph nodes on the axilae on each side and on the supraclavicular spaces. For example, before you examine the left axilla, tell the SP to rest her left arm and hand on your right arm while you are examining the axilae (the examining arm). Do the reverse for the right axilla. Note any positive or negative signs in your findings. See Table 4–12 for descriptions of probable diagnoses. Figure 4–4 is an algorithm for the diagnostic workup. See the following examples of written medical notes about the breast exam.

Breasts and Axillae

> Breasts were symmetric, no abnormalities on the skin, nipples or areolae were noted.
>
> No masses or lymph nodes on palpation. Positive watery bloody discharge on the right breast.

Breasts and Axillae

> She describes having a painless soft palpable mass, pea size, under the areolae of the left breast. No skin changes were reported. Both axilae were free of palpable nodes.

Breasts

> Are symmetric on inspection, areolas are pigmented with well formed nipple. Bilateral tenderness was detected on palpation, milky fluid was obtained on soft pressure of the nipples. No masses or other abnormalities were noted.

RESPIRATORY AND CARDIOVASCULAR SYSTEMS

Chapter 3 provides detailed information about the respiratory and cardiovascular systems.

TABLE 4–12. Breast Diseases

Fibroadenoma	Fibrocystic Disease	Page Disease	Papilloma	Cystosarcoma Phyllodes	Breast Cancer
Characteristics on Examination					
Very common; firm, smooth, round, well-defined, and extremely movable and encapsulated	The most common lesion; irregular, fibrous, rubbery tissue of some areas, cyst appearance in others	Carcinomatous disease that affects the nipple, causing pruritic/burning sensation of eczematous appearance around the nipple	Small tumors rarely palpable but often causing nipple discharge (bloody or yellowish)	A type of fibroadenoma; they are well limited without fixation and do not produce pain or nipple discharge	The most common cancer in women; palpation reveals an irregular mass that is not movable and not separable from the adjacent tissue
Age of Presentation					
Late teens to early 30s	30–50 years old	40 years or older	40 years or older	40 years or older	40–44 years old
Other					
Rapid growth during pregnancy, lactation, and premenopause	Monthly cyclic tenderness	Confused with dermatitis	Subareolar presentation	Benign tumor, but metastasis seen in 15% of cases	Risk factors very important: female gender, age older than 40 years, family history of late menopause

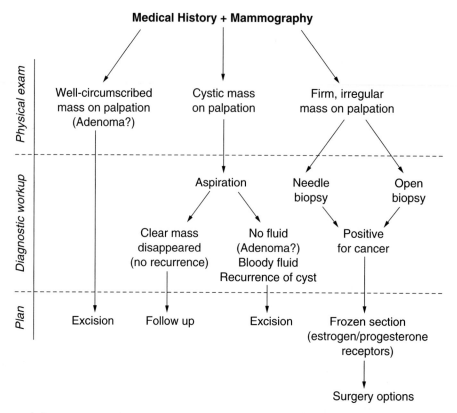

FIGURE 4–4. Diagnostic workup for the breast exam. Note: Women between 35 and 40 years of age should undergo a baseline mammogram. Women between 40 and 50 years of age should have yearly mammograms. Women with positive family histories of breast disease should be evaluated periodically and have mammograms performed as their providers prescribe. (Adapted with permission from Lawrence PF: *Essentials of General Surgery,* 2e. Philadelphia: Lippincott Williams and Wilkins, 1992, p 277.)

Abdomen

A general abdominal examination is described in Chapter 3. Remember to examine the abdomen in the correct order: inspection, auscultation, percussion, and palpation. Abdominal pain is a common complaint seen in medical practice. The characteristics of the pain, time of evolution, and the physical exam will direct you to your diagnosis. For example, acute localized abdominal pain in a woman of child-bearing age can be differentiated as indicated on Table 4–13. The clinical exam of nonpregnant women is the same as for any other patient. The abdominal exam of pregnant women is discussed in the next section.

Gynecologic-Obstetric Examination

We do not want to omit any important information that you may need during the CSA exam. Most of the information described in this section may never be presented to you by an SP on the CSA exam, but you must be prepared for any situation that you may encounter.

GYNECOLOGIC EXAMINATION

A complete abdominal examination normally occurs before the vulvar and vaginal exam. As discussed previously, you are not allowed to perform a genital exam on the CSA exam. If you suspect that a genital exam is required, indicate this in your diagnostic workup notes. Remember that good questioning about signs and symptoms and a good abdominal exam will guide your possible diagnosis and workup plans. Information re-

TABLE 4–13. Differential Diagnosis of Acute Localized Abdominal Pain in a Woman of Child-Bearing Age

Differential Diagnosis	Diagnostic Workup
1. Adnexal torsion	1. Pelvic/speculum examination
2. Acute appendicitis	2. Pregnancy test
3. Aborting intrauterine pregnancy	3. Pelvic ultrasound
4. Bleeding of corpus luteum of normal pregnancy	4. Complete blood count
5. Pelvic inflammatory disease	5. Culdocentesis
	6. Laparoscopy

garding tenderness, enlargement of the uterus, adnexa, and presence of abdominal masses will guide your findings and possible diagnosis.

Table 4–14 shows some differential diagnoses of masses found on abdominal/pelvic exam. Be prepared to react professionally and properly to any situation that may occur when you refer to the genital area in question. Be prepared if the patient is seductive or makes a sexual advance, as this is a characteristic of some seductive personalities.

OBSTETRIC EXAMINATION

Most of the information described in this section may never be presented to you on the CSA exam. Furthermore, you are not permitted to perform a cervical or vaginal exam. However, pregnant SPs can be presented, and you must be prepared to perform an appropriate abdominal exam. The physical exam includes determination of the fetal lie, presentation, and cervical examination. (These parameters are evaluated during true labor. For CSA purposes, you will never be in this real situation.) The general information that you need to obtain during the obstetric exam is as follows:

1. Uterine size.
2. Determination of lie of the fetus and presentation.
3. Fetal heart rate.
4. Vaginal exam. This helps to detect dilation, effacement, station, cervical position, and consistency of the cervix. (Although these parameters are evaluated during true labor, you are not allowed to perform a genital or vaginal exam.)

The diagnosis of labor is determined by the assessment of contractions and cervical changes. However, there are many other signs that can help to determine if the patient is in true labor (see Table 4–4). As recommended by prenatal care, after 26 weeks of gestation it is possible to perform the Leopold maneuvers (Figure 4–5). These maneu-

TABLE 4–14. Differential Diagnosis of Pelvic Masses

Differential Diagnosis	Diagnostic Workup
1. Pregnancy	1. Pelvic examination (bimanual exam)
2. Uterine leiomyoma	2. Pelvic ultrasound
3. Ovarian cyst (unruptured)	3. Pregnancy test
4. Ovarian neoplasm*	4. Complete blood count
5. Endometrioma	5. CA-125 level
6. Unruptured ectopic pregnancy	

*Consider in high-risk patients, such as those with a positive family history, history of uninterrupted ovulation such as a nulliparous woman, and women with decreased fertility, delayed childbearing, and late menopause.

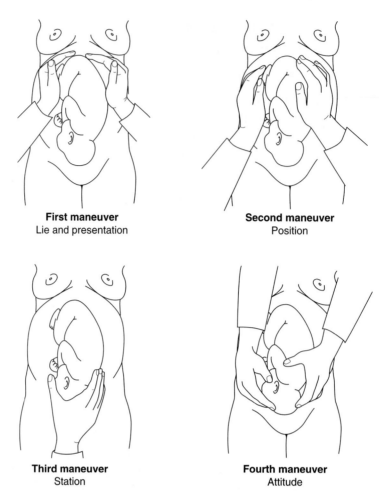

First maneuver
Lie and presentation

Second maneuver
Position

Third maneuver
Station

Fourth maneuver
Attitude

FIGURE 4–5. Leopold maneuvers and the specific aspect of fetal orientation in the uterus that can be determined. (Adapted with permission from Beckmann CR, Ling FW, Barzansky BM, et al (eds): *Obstetrics and Gynecology,* 2nd ed. Philadelphia: Lippincott Williams & Wilkins, 1995, p 171.)

vers are used to determine the fetal lie and presentation. These maneuvers are performed with both hands and while looking at the patient's face. The maneuvers are:

First maneuver. Palpate the fundus of the uterus in the maternal upper abdominal quadrants to determine on what pole it is placed. In 96% of cases, it is the breech pole.

Second maneuver. Palpate the maternal sides (right and left). This maneuver serves to determine the fetal habitus, fetal lie, and fetal position.

Third maneuver. Palpate the suprapubic region with one hand. This maneuver is useful when the presentation is totally or partially above the superior pelvic inlet and serves to determine the kind of presentation (cephalic or breech), the level of presentation, and the range of cephalic displacement if it exists. If the presentation part can be moved easily, it is said to be free; if it is not possible to move the presentation part, an engagement has occurred.

Fourth maneuver. This is only useful when the presentation part has penetrated the pelvic cavity. This maneuver is performed with both hands and looking at the feet of the patient. The purpose of this maneuver is the same as the third maneuver.

Detailed information about normal labor and delivery can be reviewed in gynecology and obstetrics textbooks. See the following written notes for examples of obstetric exam notes. Not all the information in these examples necessarily reflects a situation seen on the CSA exam.

Obstetric Exam (Ob/Gyn)

Uterine size: 20 cm, FHR: 140/min, Quickening +

Leopold's maneuver revealed a longitudinal lie position and occiput presentation. Cervical exam reveal 0 dilation, firm in consistency, posterior position.

Obstetric Exam (Ob/Gyn)

Uterine size: 35 cm, FHR 100/min

Leopold's revealed a longitudinal lie position with breech presentation. Cervical exam showed 6 cm dilation, 80% effaced, station +1.

Gynecologic Exam (Ob/Gyn)

Tenderness on palpation of lower abdomen. A 10 cm well circumscribed mass was detected on the left side on bimanual exam. Three nabotian cysts were observed on cervix. No other abnormalities found.

Ob/Gyn Exam (Ob/Gyn)

Uterine size 25 cm; FHR 120/min.

Leopold's revealed a longitudinal lie position with occiput presentation. The low abdominal exam was unremarkable. Vaginal exam reveals small cluster of painful vesicles on the right labia, similar lesions were observed on the cervix.

Other

Depending on the case presented, you can add information about other organs and/or systems that you consider relevant. The clinical exam of a pregnant patient cannot be considered complete without examining the extremities, looking for signs of varices and edema and checking reflexes. Edema always alerts you to the possibility of fluid retention and then the presence of preeclampsia. Edema is usually detected during routing prenatal visits. Increases more than 0.5 kg/wk are abnormal. Any edema seen above the knees that does not disappear after 12 hours of bedrest is also abnormal. Examining the reflexes is also important because hyperreflexia is a sign of severe preeclampsia (Table 4–15).

URINARY INCONTINENCE AND PELVIC RELAXATION

Urinary incontinence (UI) is a common complaint that affects 25 million Americans. UI is more common in white multiparous women and is rare in black and Asian women. Other risk factors include problems that increase intraabdominal pressure such as chronic cough, straining, ascites, and large pelvic tumors. Symptoms can be feelings of heaviness, pelvic pressure, dyspareunia, increase in frequency and urgency, urinary incontinence, or no symptoms at all. Table 4–16 lists a differential diagnosis for patients with these symptoms. The possible diagnosis and initial tentative diagnosis should be explained to the SP. Remember that the initial management of urinary incontinence includes pelvic exercises (Kegel exercises), weight reduction, and control of cough or infection.

DIFFERENTIAL DIAGNOSIS

You should limit the number of differential diagnoses to five. Review different examples in this book.

TABLE 4–15. Hypertension in Pregnancy

Preeclampsia	HELLP syndrome	Eclampsia	Gestational HTN	Chronic HTN
HTN with proteinuria, edema, or both induced by pregnancy after the 20th week (unless it is a molar pregnancy)	Subcategory of preeclampsia in which patients present with **h**emolytic anemia, **el**evated **l**iver enzymes, and **l**ow **p**latelets	Presence of convulsions in a woman who meets the criteria of preeclampsia	HTN during the latter half of pregnancy or during the first 24 hours after delivery; patient has no criteria for preeclampsia, and the condition disappears in 10 days	The presence of persistent HTN before the 20th week of pregnancy in the absence of hydatiform mole

General Diagnostic Workup Plan

1. Renal studies: urinalysis, 24-hr urinary protein, 24-hr urinary volume, BUN/Cr
2. Liver function tests: AST, ALT, total bilirubin
3. Complete blood count (platelets)
4. Peripheral blood smear
5. Lactate dehydrogenase

AST = aspartate aminotransferase; ALT = alanine aminotransferase; BUN = blood urea nitrogen; Cr = creatinine; HTN = hypertension.

DIAGNOSTIC WORKUP

There are several routine tests and procedures that you need to order or consider in a pregnant woman. Some tests are ordered in a routine fashion depending on the stage of pregnancy. Others will be ordered depending on the patient's situation. The same indications as in the general written notes apply here. Limit yourself to five diagnostic workups. Diagnostic workups can be diagnostic tests or procedures (see Table 4–3).

TABLE 4–16. Differential Diagnosis of a Patient with Symptoms Related to Pelvic Relaxation

Differential Diagnosis	Diagnostic Workup
1. Pelvic relaxation (cystocele, rectocele, urethrocele, enterocele, uterine prolapse)	1. Standing stress test*
2. Urinary incontinence (stress, urge, total, and overflow)	2. Pelvic examination
3. Urinary tract infection	3. Cotton swab test†
4. Pelvic tumors	4. Urinalysis
	5. Urinary culture
	6. Pelvic ultrasound

*Ask the patient to stand over a towel with her legs apart (the patient should not be wearing underwear). Then ask her to cough. Observe if any urine appears on the towel.
†Serves to detect the hypermobility of the bladder neck. The normal bladder neck motion on straining is less than 30°.

5

Nervous System: Writing Medical Notes

INTRODUCTION

The neurologic exam is performed under the general medical history format, as covered in Chapter 3.

How do you approach a standardized patient (SP) having a neurologic consultation? Your approach will depend on the case presented to you. For example, in a young, healthy individual, a simple screening neurologic exam is more than sufficient, and the findings can be mentioned in your general written medical notes if you consider it pertinent. For an older patient, a more detailed neurologic exam will probably be necessary as part of the general exam. In addition, if the SP has a neurologic problem, you will need to focus your questions and explore this area. For all these reasons, you need to know neuroanatomy and neurophysiology well to perform an excellent clinical exam.

The following section is a brief review of the normal and broad physioanatomic aspects in relation to the clinical exam. Clinical findings will be correlated with pathognomonic clinical syndromes that you may encounter during the CSA exam. For more information about any specific case related to neuroanatomy or neurophysiology, refer to detailed textbooks in the appropriate areas.

REVIEW OF THE NERVOUS SYSTEM: ANATOMY AND PHYSIOLOGY

Your knowledge of normal anatomy and physiology will always help you successfully assess your patient. The nervous system can be divided into three groups, which have overlapping functions:

Sensory functions
Integrative functions
Motor functions

Together these functions help us keep in touch with the environment and maintain homeostasis, thought processes, learning, and memory. Millions of sensory receptors throughout the body detect changes (**stimuli**) in and out of the nervous system. The external receptors detect variables such as temperature, light, and sound. The internal receptors detect changes in blood pressure, pH, electrolytes, and CO_2 concentration. All the information gathered is called **sensory input.** The sensory input is converted into electrical signals (**nerve impulses**) that are transmitted to the brain. These signals are brought together to stimulate the production of exocrine or endocrine secretions, to produce thoughts, or to be added to the memory. Decisions are made each moment based on sensory input, and this constitutes the integration of the nervous system. The nervous system responds to sensory input and integration by sending signals to muscles (e.g., causing them to contract) or to glands (e.g., causing them to secrete substances). This is known as efferent output or motor function.

The Reflex Arc

The **neuron** is the structural unit of the nervous system, and the **reflex arc** is the functional unit. The reflex arc is an involuntary response that occurs following a change either outside or inside the body. A reflex can be elicited by external stimuli such as heat, pain (e.g., when an injection is given), or stretching a muscle or tendon (e.g., when using a hammer). The reflex arc is a type of conduction pathway. The most common reflex response consists of two neurons, but there can be three or more neurons in a conduction pathway. Reflexes are necessary to maintain homeostasis. An intact reflex response involves the integrity of the following:

1. Special sensory endings in the muscle
2. Sensory nerve fibers (afferent impulse)
3. Motor neuron (the anterior horn cell)
4. Motor anterior root (efferent impulse)
5. Neuromuscular junction
6. Functional muscle fibers

Some reflexes are superficial or cutaneous; this not only depends on their spinal reflex arc, but also on their pathways to and from the cerebral cortex (Figure 5–1). The reflex arc is used by clinicians to determine the integrity of the nervous system.

Nervous System Divisions

Figure 5–2 is a commonly used classification of the nervous system. A very simple way to classify the central nervous system (CNS) anatomically is to say that the CNS is "everything that is inside the bones" (i.e., skull and vertebrae).

Motor Pathways

Motor pathways are also known as **descending pathways.** There are three major tracts that descend to the anterior horn cells. All of these pathways regulate motor activity and only through the lower motor neurons (despite the appearance of nerve impulses

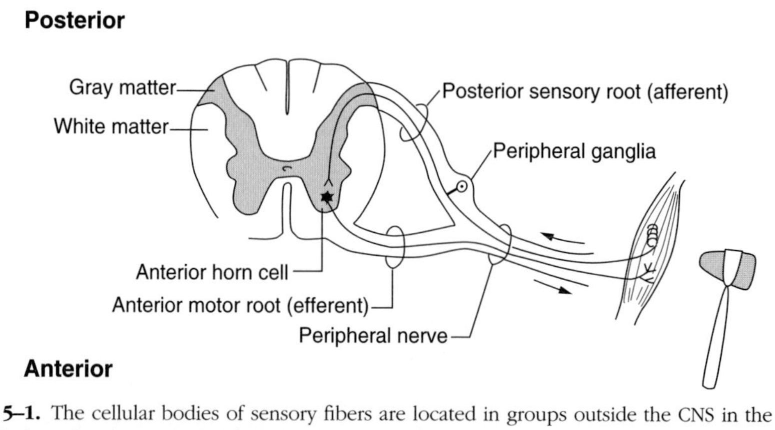

FIGURE 5–1. The cellular bodies of sensory fibers are located in groups outside the CNS in the peripheral ganglia. (Adapted with permission from Fix JD: *High-Yield Neuroanatomy,* 2nd ed. Philadelphia: Lippincott Williams & Wilkins, 2000, p 36.)

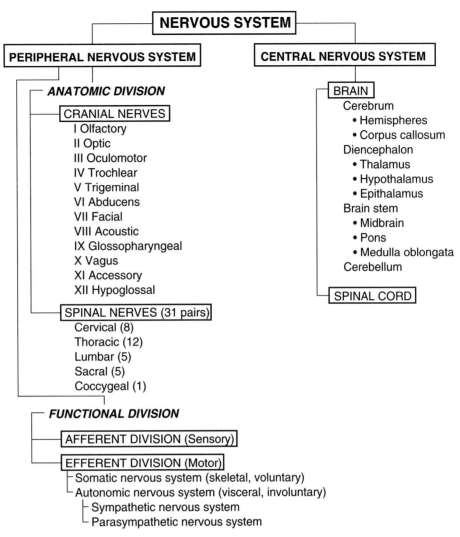

FIGURE 5–2. Classification of the nervous system.

on the motor cortex, basal ganglia, or reflex in the sensory receptor). These pathways are the corticospinal tract (pyramidal tract), corticobulbar tract, extrapyramidal tract, and cerebellar system.

CORTICOSPINAL TRACT (PYRAMIDAL TRACT)

The fibers in this pathway transmit impulses from the cerebral cortex to the spinal cord and provide voluntary movement, which is transmitted through the motor fibers traveling down from the motor cortex through the internal capsule. Most of them (90%) cross to the opposite side of the cord at the **medulla oblongata** level and then continue down in the spinal cord, where they synapse with the anterior horn cells or with intermediate neurons. This tract not only coordinates voluntary movements, but also participates in the integration of highly skilled motor function by stimulation or inhibition.

CORTICOBULBAR TRACT

This tract is similar to the corticospinal fibers that are connected with the motor nerve cells. The fibers in this pathway transmit impulses from the cerebral motor cortex to the cranial nerves (CNs) nuclei (of CN V, CN VI, CN VII, CN IX, CN X, CN XI, and CN XII) located in the pons and the medulla oblongata. Like the corticospinal tract, corticobulbar tract fibers travel down through the internal capsule and most of them cross to the opposite side. Both corticospinal and corticobulbar neurons are called upper motor neurons.

EXTRAPYRAMIDAL TRACT

This complex motor system helps maintain muscle tone and control gross automatic movements, such as walking and maintaining posture and balance. This system includes pathways from the cerebral cortex, basal ganglia, brain stem, and spinal cord.

CEREBELLAR SYSTEM

The cerebellum coordinates voluntary and involuntary movements to produce smooth muscle movements, thus preventing jerking and trembling motions. This system receives both sensory and motor input, coordinates muscular activity, maintains equilibrium, and helps control posture. When it is damaged, movements such as running, walking, writing, and maintaining posture become impaired.

Sensory Pathways

Sensory pathways are known as **ascending pathways.** As described previously, sensory impulses do not only participate in reflex activity, but they also give rise to conscious sensation. The sensation initiated in any receptor on skin, tendon, muscle, or viscera travels along a sensory nerve fiber (**peripheral nerve**) toward the spinal cord. The sensory nerve fiber follows the posterior dorsal root; immediately after entry into the spinal cord, it enters either the posterior columns or the spinothalamic tract.

POSTERIOR COLUMNS

The posterior columns carry sensations of **position, vibration,** and **fine touch** (with accurate localization). The fibers conducting the sensations of position and vibration pass directly into the posterior columns and travel upward to the upper cervical spinal cord and medulla region, where they synapse with *secondary sensory neurons.* These secondary neurons cross over to the other side, where they continue to the thalamus.

SPINOTHALAMIC TRACT

The spinothalamic tract carries sensations of **pain, temperature,** and **crude touch** (without accurate localization). Within one or two spinal segments from their entry into the spinal cord, fibers conducting the sensations of pain and temperature pass into the posterior horn and synapse with "*secondary sensory neurons*." These neurons cross to the opposite side just anterior to the central canal and pass upward in the lateral spinothalamic tract to the thalamus.

Touch impulses originating on one side of the body travel up both sides of the cord. Touch sensation is often preserved despite any partial damage to the spinal cord. The thalamus serves as a relay station for sensory impulses, except for smell. For full perception, a third group of sensory neurons carries the impulses from synapses in the thalamus to the sensory cortex of the brain, where discriminations are made. Lesions at different points in the sensory pathways produce different kinds of sensory loss. Knowledge of **dermatomes** will help you localize peripheral nerve lesions (Figure 5–3).

NERVOUS SYSTEM MEDICAL HISTORY

The following format table represents only a general description of the neurologic exam (Figure 5–4). Use this format to organize your ideas to perform the pertinent maneuvers during the clinical exam.

A great amount of data concerning the nervous system (e.g., speech, mental status,

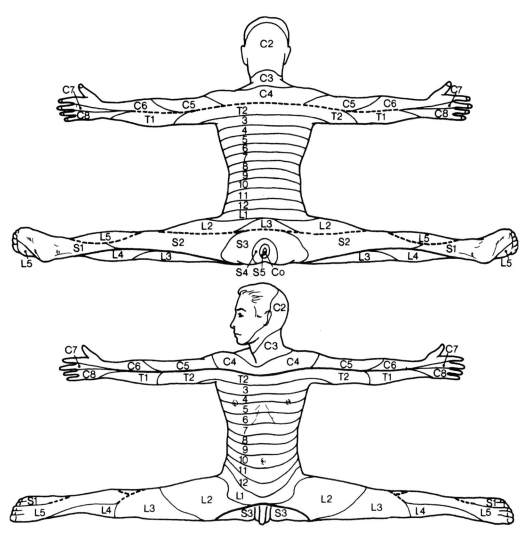

FIGURE 5–3. Normal dermatome distribution. (Reprinted with permission from Haymaker W, Woodhall B: *Peripheral Nerve Injuries,* 2nd ed. Philadelphia: WB Saunders, 1952, p 32.)

evaluation of some cranial nerves) is frequently obtained during the initial interview or during the general clinical exam. It is important to remember that the medical history and physical exam are performed as part of the general clinical exam (see Chapter 3). When possible, neurologic written notes should be recorded in the same format as general written notes. For CSA purposes, your own criteria are important in selecting the most relevant information for the written note.

A) COMPLETE NEUROLOGIC EXAMINATION	**B) MENINGEAL TESTS**
1. Mental status examination and speech	1. Kernig test
2. Cranial nerves examination	2. Brudzinski test
3. Motor system examination: *tone, strength, coordination*	
4. Sensory system examination	
5. Reflexes examination	

FIGURE 5–4. General format of a neurologic exam.

Complete Neurologic Examination

You will have to perform a complete neurologic exam on an SP who requires it. Focus appropriately on this area without forgetting to examine other organs and systems. The neurologic exam must be performed whenever possible under the general format of a patient note (see Figure 3–1).

MENTAL STATUS EXAMINATION (MSE) AND SPEECH

The mental status examination (MSE) and general evaluation of speech should be done in the context of the interview and in the context of the general medical history and physical exam. During your conversation with the SP, you should evaluate his or her level of consciousness, paying special attention to grooming, orientation, personal hygiene, facial expression, mood, affection, speech, and memory. Note if the patient's vocabulary is in the context of his or her culture and level of education. As you talk with the SP, you can get a rough estimate of the SP's intelligence. Screen the patient quickly to assess **attention, memory,** and **orientation** (specifically, awareness of time, place, and other people; you can document as *well oriented X3*). Write down any abnormality in speech.

The MSE exam can be used in different situations and for different patients. This test is not exclusive of the nervous system exam. If you know it well and consider it necessary, you can perform the Mini Mental Status Exam (MMSE) to quantify your evaluation of cognitive and intellectual functions. For many patients, this evaluation is sufficient and serves as a screening of mental status. However, if you believe that your patient has a neuropsychiatric problem, you may have to perform a psychiatric examination.

CRANIAL NERVES

CNs are susceptible to disorders that are particular to them. These disorders rarely affect spinal nerves. The cranial nerves (CN) are explored alone or in groups according to their function.

CN I: Olfactory Nerve

Examine one nostril at a time. Ask the patient to close his or her eyes and then to identify a substance that you present; you can use coffee, tobacco, soap, or pepper. This test is not performed routinely, but must be done when the patient refers to loss of taste or smell. Hyposmia or bilateral anosmia could be caused by nasal infections, pernicious anemia, normal aging, excessive smoking, or cocaine use. For pernicious anemia, the diagnostic workup should include (1) complete blood count (CBC) (hemoglobin/hematocrit [Hb/Hct]), mean corpuscular volume (MCV); (2) peripheral blood smear; (3) lactate dehydrogenase (LDH), serum vitamin B_{12}, and folate levels; (4) serum methylmalonic acid (MMA) + homocysteine; and (5) Shilling test; also be alert for other neurologic findings. Unilateral loss of smell without nasal disease could suggest a lesion involving the inferior aspect of the frontal lobe. Hallucinatory smells are presented during partial complex seizures. During the CSA exam, you might not have the material to perform the clinical exam of this cranial nerve, but you need to be prepare to do it if the situation mandates, or indicate it on your diagnostic workup plan in the medical note.

CN II: Optic Nerve

The discrimination of fine colors and visual details depends basically on an intact optic nerve and intact pathways to the occipital cortex. A lesion on the optic nerve causes a decrease in visual perception. An abnormal pupillary reaction to light indicates a lesion in the optic nerve. When the affected eye is stimulated by light, the response *decreases* significantly but response *increases* in the normal eye. Examination of the optic nerve proceeds as follows.

VISUAL ACUITY TEST   Use a Snellen Eye Chart if you have one in the examining room and if it is indicated by the history. At this time, there is no comment by CSA test takers about the Snellen Eye Chart in the CSA exam rooms. However, being prepared for any situation is the key to success.

Ask the SP to *cover one eye* while wearing his or her glasses. The patient should be 20 ft (6 m) away from the chart (approximately 6 steps). Ask the patient to read the letters on the chart, starting with the largest one and progressing to the smallest. Identify the smallest line of print that the SP is able to read the best (i.e., the SP can read more than half the letters on the line). Document visual acuity as designated at the side of this line, expressed as the fraction that appears to the side of the letters (e.g., 20/40 [the numerator indicates the distance in feet from the patient to the chart; the denominator indicates the distance in feet from which a normal eye can read the line of letters]. The normal average for the visual acuity test is 20/20 ft or 6/6 m. If the SP cannot identify the biggest letter (20/200) on the chart, he or she can move close to the chart until the letter can be identified. In such a case, the numerator will be modified (e.g., 10/60 or 15/200). If the patient still cannot see the letters, hold up one or two fingers and ask the patient to count them. If the patient cannot see your fingers, ask him or her to recognize your moving hand.

When a patient can only recognize the light from a flashlight, ask him or her to let you know in what visual field the light is seen (nasal field, temporal field). In the **myopic eye** the anterior-posterior diameter of the eye is increased in comparison to the normal eye; these patient are **nearsighted.** During the funduscopic examination, you will use longer focus lenses in the ophthalmoscope, with a minus **diopter.** Diopters are the units of refracting power of lenses, denoting the reciprocal of the focal length expressed in meters. In the **hyperopic eye,** the anterior-posterior diameter of the eye is diminished; these patients are **farsighted.** During the funduscopic examination, you will use shorter focus lenses, with a plus diopter.

Diseases of the optic nerve can cause monocular blindness, central scotomas, poor perception of colors, and blurred vision. If the lesion is severe, it is possible that the patient may not be able to distinguish between darkness and brightness. With a moderate lesion, the central scotoma can be described as a tangential screen when the patient tries to read. With mild to moderate unilateral lesions, the defect may be manifested only by a loss of visual acuity and a decrease in color perception.

VISUAL FIELDS BY CONFRONTATION   It is important to bear in mind the normal anatomy of the optic pathway and its abnormalities when performing the clinical exam (Figure 5–5). Place yourself in front of the patient (1 or 2 ft away) so that your face will be directly in front and on the level with his or her face. Ask the SP to close one eye and look at the patient's eyes directly. Then close your eye that is directly opposite of the patient's closed eye. Use a pen or pencil to check the visual fields by moving to the sides of his or her visual fields and asking the patient to respond the moment the object is detected. Compare the SP's responses with your own visual field. Repeat the same maneuver with the other eye.

A healthy person looking straight to the front is able to see a moving object almost 90% to the side. Visual field defects that you may find during this clinical exam include the presence of scotoma. **Scotoma** is an absence of vision in one area of the visual field. Based on this definition, hemianopsia is a scotoma in the half part and quadrantanopia is a scotoma in one quadrant of the visual field, respectively.

Only the central portions of the two visual fields are binocular; the temporal margins are monocular. Both temporal sides need to be stimulated at the same time to detect mild hemianopic lesions of the optic pathway or cortex. Common visual fields defects are as follows:

1. **Monocular blindness.** This indicates a lesion in the optic nerve anterior to the optic chiasm. Causes include amaurosis fugax as well as central vein and artery retinal occlusion (see Figure 5–5).

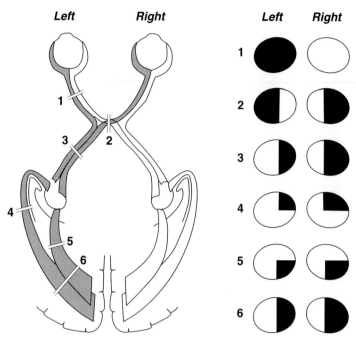

FIGURE 5–5. The optic pathway and its lesions. *Lesion 1* represents monocular blindness. *Lesion 2* represents bitemporal hemianopsia. *Lesion 3* represents homonymous hemianopsias. *Lesion 4* represents upper homonymous quadrantanopsias. *Lesion 5* represents lower homonymous quadrantanopsias. *Lesion 6* represents homonymous hemianopsia. (Adapted with permission from Fix JD: *High-Yield Neuroanatomy,* 2nd ed. Philadelphia: Lippincott Williams & Wilkins, 2000, p 91.)

2. **Bitemporal hemianopsia.** This indicates a lesion at the optic chiasm. Causes may include pituitary tumor, meningioma, or craniopharyngioma tumor (see Figure 5–5).

3. **Homonymous hemianopsias.** This indicates a lesion behind the optic chiasm usually in the optic tract, optic radiation, or cerebral cortex. This lesion affects the temporal side of one visual field and the nasal visual field of the other eye. In Figure 5–5, numbers 3 and 6 indicate a **right homonymous hemianopsia.**

4. **Upper homonymous quadrantanopsias.** This indicates a lesion of the optic radiation in the temporal lobe (Meyer loop) and involves only a portion of the nerve fibers (see Figure 5–5).

5. **Lower homonymous quadrantanopsias.** This indicates a lesion of the optic radiations in the parietal lobe.

6. **Right homonymous hemianopsia.** This indicates a complete interruption of fibers in the optic radiation. The visual defect is similar to that produced by a lesion of the optic tract (see Figure 5–5).

Finally, for the CSA exam, if you find a patient has any of the above problems, be prepared to order a **perimetric examination of the visual fields** in your diagnostic workup plan. In real clinical practice, you would refer this patient to an ophthalmologist; for the CSA, you are not allowed to order referrals on your medical notes.

OPHTHALMOSCOPIC EXAMINATION   Ask the patient to look straight ahead. If the patient wears glasses with a substantial correction, perform the funduscopic examination with the patient wearing the glasses. Find the correct lens and then focus on the optic disc, review its color and shape, and then proceed to examine the vessels. The arteries are narrower than the veins and have a brighter color. The retinal veins pulsate in 80%–90% of patients (which indirectly indicates that the CSF is at normal pressure).

The fundus can be divided into quadrants to help you in the localization of any abnormal finding (such as exudates or hemorrhage). Draw imaginary horizontal and vertical lines that cross through the fovea, thereby yielding the superior temporal, inferior temporal, inferior nasal, and superior nasal quadrants (Figure 5–6). Furthermore, you can name the fundus horizontally as 3 o'clock and 9 o'clock and vertically as 12 o'clock and 6 o'clock, respectively. In your notes, mention the specific quadrant in which there is an abnormal finding; if pertinent, draw a diagram. Figure 5–6 shows a normal fundoscopy and diagram.

Also look for:

1. **Normal optic disk.** The optic disk is a yellowish-orange to creamy pink oval structure. Normally you will note that the vessels (arteries and veins) converge at the center of the optic disk.
2. **Papilledema.** This often occurs without visual complaints and is best seen with a red-free light in plus lenses. The vessels seen are tortuous; loss of vein pulsations, flame hemorrhages, and hyperemic and cotton wool spots are seen. There is also a loss of disc borders. Bilateral papilledema is a sign of cranial hypertension. Unilateral papilledema can be seen in optic neuritis and in ischemic neuropathy.
3. **Optic atrophy.** This process appears after damage to the ganglion cells or axons found between the retinal nerve layer and the lateral geniculate body. The presence of papilledema in one eye and optic disk atrophy in the other is known as Foster Kennedy syndrome, frequently related to a meningioma of the sphenoid bone in the side of the atrophy.

It is important to remember that the ophthalmoscopic examination forms part of the evaluation of every patient. Patients with hypertension and diabetics require an ophthalmoscopic evaluation. Important differential diagnoses to consider during an ophthalmoscopic examination are shown in Table 5–1.

CN III, CN IV, and CN VI: Oculomotor, Trochlear, and Abducens Nerves

These cranial nerves are studied together, because all of them innervate the **extraocular muscles.** The CN III pair also innervates the pupillary sphincter, the eyelid elevator muscle, and the muscle of the ciliary body.

EXTRAOCULAR MUSCLES (EOM)   Any damage to these muscles, nerves, or their respective nuclei on the midbrain can cause double or blurred vision. If an SP has **pto-**

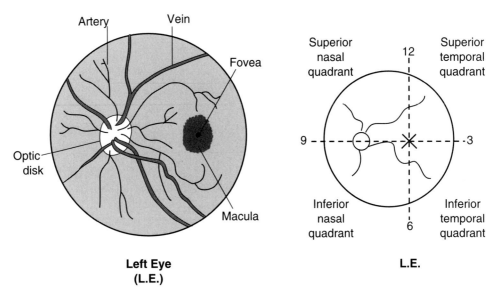

FIGURE 5–6. Normal fundoscopy and diagram.

TABLE 5–1. Differential Diagnosis to Consider During an Ophthalmoscopic Examination

Retinal Vascular Disease	Optic Nerve Disease	Chiasmatic Lesions	Optic Tract/Radiation Geniculate/Occipital
Retinal artery and vein occlusion	Optic neuritis*	Meningioma	Tumors
Hypertensive retinopathy	Arteritic optic neuropathy (due to temporal arteritis)	Pituitary tumors	Stroke
Diabetic retinopathy		Craniopharyngioma	
Blood dyscrasias (thrombocytopenia, severe anemia, and sickle cell disease)	Nonarteritic optic neuro-pathy (due to hyper-tension)		
	Tumors		
Diagnostic Workup			
1. EKG	1. MRI	1. Lateral skull radiographs	1. CT scan
2. Chest radiographs	2. Evoked potentials	2. MRI	2. MRI
3. Doppler ultrasound of carotid arteries	3. LP	3. Prolactin	
4. Angiography	4. ESR	4. TSH, T$_4$	
5. CT scan/MRI		5. Serum hCG	
6. CBC		6. Pregnancy test	
7. PT, PTT			
8. ESR			
9. Electrolyte and glucose levels			

CBC = complete blood count; CT = computed tomography; EKG = electrocardiogram; ESR = erythrocyte sedimentation rate; hCG = human chorionic gonadotropin; LP = lumbar puncture; MRI = magnetic resonance imaging; PT = prothrombin time; PTT = partial thromboplastin time; T$_4$ = thyroxine; TIA = transient ischemic attack; TSH = thyroid-stimulating hormone.
*Optic neuritis is associated with demyelinative diseases such as multiple sclerosis, infectious diseases such as varicella zoster infection, and autoimmune disorders such as systemic lupus erythematosus. Loss of vision can suddenly develop and can be associated with eye movement disorders.

sis, find out whether the problem is bilateral or unilateral. If the SP has **diplopia,** ask if covering one (any) eye (binocular diplopia) relieves the problem. Monocular diplopia results from abnormality in one eye (crystalline dislocation, corneal diseases). Diplopia will disappear only when the SP covers the affected eye. Then ask the SP to mention how the images are. If it is horizontal or vertical, if it increases to one direction, and if it is constant or intermittent. Assess the EOM movements by telling the SP to follow your finger or pencil as you move on the six cardinal fields of gaze. Always inspect for the normal **conjugate** or parallel movements of the eyes in each direction or any abnormal deviation. Note the presence of any abnormal movements such as nystagmus or oscillatory movements. Individual ocular nerve lesions include the following:

CN III lesion. This can present with ptosis and deviation of the eye down and outward with or without pupillary dilation. Pupillary dilation is seen more frequently in association with aneurysms and herniations. Other causes of oculomotor nerve palsy include meningitis, tumor, infarction, carotid aneurysm, carotid cavernous fistula, cavernous sinus thrombosis, and herpes zoster.
CN IV lesion. This causes the patient to be unable to move the eye downward and inward. The head is frequently tilted. This is a common cause of symptomatic vertical diplopia. The paralysis of the superior oblique muscle results in extortion and weakness of downward movement. Isolated trochlear nerve palsy can occurs because of the same causes as those for oculomotor nerve palsy, with the exception of aneurysm.
CN VI lesion. In this case, the patient is unable to abduct the paretic eye. The affected eye deviates medially in the direction of the opposing muscle. Unilateral or bilateral abducens palsy is a classic sign of increased intracranial pressure (ICP). The diagnosis can be confirmed

if papilledema is observed on fundus examination. Other causes include infarcts, tumors, hemorrhages, vascular malformation, and multiple sclerosis.

These three cranial nerves are frequently affected at the same time. CN III and CN VI are affected frequently, and the principal cause of motor paresis includes aneurysm and diabetes. In addition to ICP, Wernicke-Korsakoff syndrome may be a cause of CN VI pair paresis. **Wernicke encephalopathy** is characterized by ataxia, confusion, and ophthalmoplegia. **Korsakoff psychosis** is characterized by amnesia and confabulation. The cause of this syndrome is thiamine deficiency, which is commonly seen in alcoholics. For other organic brain syndromes, differential diagnoses must be made. The general diagnostic workup plan in these patients includes computed tomography (CT) scan of the head, glucose, measurement of electrolyte levels, and complete blood count (CBC).

PUPILLARY REFLEXES   Take note of the size, shape, and symmetry of the pupils. Test the pupillary reaction to light and to accommodation and review the pupil types (Table 5–2).

1. **Reaction to light.** Ask the patient to look into the distance, then illuminate one eye (pupil) with the penlight and check for constriction in the same eye and pupillary constriction on the opposite eye (consensual reaction).
2. **Pupillary reaction to accommodation.** Ask the patient to look into the distance, then put your finger 8–10 cm in front of him or her and check for bilateral pupillary constriction and convergence of the eyes.

TABLE 5–2. Pupil Types

Anisocoria	Small Fixed Pupils	Dilated Fixed Pupils	Horner Syndrome Pupil	Argyll Robertson Pupil	Tonic Pupil	Oculomotor paralysis
Describes subtle inequality in pupil size, up to 0.5 mm	Bilateral small fixed pupil (pinpoint pupils)	Bilateral dilated and fixed pupils that react slowly to light	Miosis Ptosis Good response to light Anhidrosis	Small, irregular pupils No response to light Good constriction during accommodation	Pupil dilated and fixed in bright light Constriction occurs slowly on constant stimulation	Dilated pupil that reacts neither to light nor accommodation
Association						
It should be found in normal subjects. If it is important, it may indicate sympathetic paresis or palsy.	Opioid use or abuse Miotic drugs, such as pilocarpine In comatose patient, consider pontine hemorrhage	It results from use of antimuscarinic agents, such as amobarbital, sedatives, (e.g., glutethimide), or mushroom poisoning	Tumorous or inflammatory involvement of cervical lymph nodes Surgical or other neck trauma Neoplastic invasion of proximal part of brachial plexus	Neurosyphilis	Called Homes-Adie syndrome when accompanied by lack of response of deep tendon reflexes	Could be associated with deviation of the eye laterally and downward

CN V: Trigeminal Nerve

The trigeminal nerve has three divisions: CN V1 (**ophthalmic**), CN V2 (**maxillary**), and CN V3 (**mandibular**). All three divisions are sensory. Their cutaneus distribution is shown in Figure 5–7. Each of the three divisions provides the sensory component to an autonomic ganglion. The motor portion of the nerve innervates (CN V3) the ipsilateral muscles of mastication and a few other muscles.

The clinical exam of this cranial nerve can be approached as follows.

MOTOR EXPLORATION   Ask the patient to open and close his or her jaw and **make movements to the sides.** Note any muscle wasting. Assess the power of the masseter and temporalis muscles by resisting the SP's attempts at opening and closing the jaw. While palpating the masseter muscles, ask the patient to clench the teeth. Repeat the same maneuver while palpating the temporal muscle. Note the strength of the muscle contraction. When **motor paresis** exists (and when unilateral paresis of CN XII exists), the tongue and the jaw suffer a deviation to the side of the lesion.

SENSORY EXAM   This section describes the sensory examination of the face and cornea. Start the exam by asking the patient to close his or her eyes. Then test the forehead, cheeks, and jaw for tactile or pain sensation. You can use a pin while you stimulate the skin of the face bilaterally and ask the patient to report whether it is a *dull* or *sharp* pain. The **Corneal reflex test** can be performed by using a fine wisp of cotton and asking the patient to look upward. Then touch the cornea (not the conjunctiva) lightly, checking to see if the patient's eye blinks (the normal reaction carried out by this nerve). Any abnormality will be referred to as a loss of or diminished sensation. Table 5–3 lists some facial sensation disorders and their possible causes. An irritative lesion, such as trigeminal neuralgia, more frequently affects the mandibular and maxillary roots and is characterized by intense paroxysmal pain in those regions without the loss of sensitivity.

CN VII: Facial Nerve

The seventh cranial nerve is mainly a motor nerve supplying all muscles concerned with facial expression on one side. The sensory component is small. The anterior two thirds of the tongue is the sensorial component of this nerve and it controls the ability to taste. During the patient interview, note any alteration in facial expression as well as any asymmetry, tics, or other abnormal movements. During the clinical exam, ask the patient to raise the eyebrows and then frown, show his or her teeth, smile, and puff (i.e., hold air in cheeks). Tell the patient to close his or her eyes tightly so that you cannot

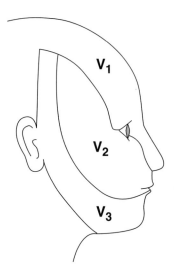

FIGURE 5–7. Trigeminal nerve (CN V) innervation.

TABLE 5–3. Facial Sensory Disorders and Their Possible Causes.

Motor-Sensory Disorders: Trigeminal Neuropathy	Pure Pain Disorder (Sensory): Trigeminal Neuralgia*
Characteristics	
Most patients present with sensory loss on the face or with weakness of the jaw muscles. Lesions of the cavernous sinus can affect the CN V1 division. CN V1 and CN V2 lesions as well as lesions of the superior fissure can affect the CN V1 division. CN V1 affection causes corneal anesthesia with increased risk of ulceration.	This disorder occurs in middle-aged and elderly persons (50 years of age and older) Affects women more commonly then men. Signs and symptoms include excruciating paroxysm of pain in the lips, gums, cheek or chin. Tactile trigger zones exist and exacerbate attacks.
Etiology	
Tumors of the middle cranial fossa (meningiomas)	CN V microneuroma
Trigeminal nerve schwannomas	Compression by aneurysm or tumor
Metastatic tumors	Relation with diabetes, multiple sclerosis, and trauma
Differential Diagnosis	
Lateral medullary syndrome	Dental problems
Sensory involvement with thalamic, capsular, or cortical infarction.	Sinusitis
Tetanus (trismus)	Temporomandibular joint disease
Phenothiazine drugs (adverse effect)	Cluster headaches
Temporomandibular joint disease	Diabetes
	Multiple sclerosis

General Diagnostic Workup Plan

1. CT head scan
2. Sinus x-ray series
3. MRI arteriograms
4. Lumbar puncture
5. CBC, electrolytes
6. Glucose

CBC = complete blood count; CT − computed tomography; MRI = magnetic resonance imaging
*Also known as idiopathic trigeminal neuralgia, or tic douloureux.

open them. To examine taste, tell the patient to close his or her eyes and protrude the tongue. Place a concentrated solution of vinegar, sugar, or salt on the tongue and ask the patient to identify the substance (Note: This function is not normally tested).

This nerve can be affected in different sections of its pathway. Superior face muscles are innervated by neurons from both sides of the motor cortex. Right frontal and orbicularis oculi muscles are innervated by CN VII fibers, and the nuclear cell bodies located in the anterior horn receive corticopontine fibers from the right and left motor cortex areas. Inferior face muscles are innervated by neurons from the CN VII nucleus, which receives impulses only from the opposite cerebral cortex (left cortex). Therefore, unilateral left cortical lesions do not alter the function of the orbicular and frontal right muscles, although orbicularis ori and platysma myoides muscles will be affected. Unilateral upper motor neuron lesions only produce facial weakness in the inferior region.

A complete interruption of the facial nerve at the stylomastoid foramen paralyzes all muscles of facial expression of the affected side (superior and inferior muscles). The corner of the mouth drops and the skin folds are effaced, the forehead is wrinkled, the palpebral fissure is widened, and the eyelids will not close. When closing the eyelids is attempted, both eyes roll upward (**Bell phenomenon**).

In lesions in the facial canal above the junction with the chorda tympani but below the geniculate ganglion, all symptoms described previously appear in addition to loss of taste over the anterior two thirds of the tongue on the same side. **Hyperacusis** exists if the nerve of the stapedius muscle is involved. **Lacrimation** is reduced if the geniculate ganglion or the motor root proximal to it is involved. Lesions at this level may affect the adjacent eighth nerve, causing deafness, tinnitus, or dizziness. Intrapontine lesions that paralyze the face often affect the abducens nucleus and the corticospinal sensory tracts. If peripheral paralysis has existed for some time and motor function has begun but is incomplete, a kind of contracture may appear.

Always remember to ask the patient if he or she has noted any loss of taste on the front part of the tongue, if there have been any strange sounds in the ear in the same side of the paresis, and if there is excessive tearing of the eye on the same side. Table 5–4 lists the diverse localization and etiology of facial nerve lesions. Table 5–5 provides a concise explanation of Bell palsy and its differential diagnosis.

Finally, percuss the top of the check just below the zygomatic bone or in the front of the ear, trying to elicit a positive **Chvostek sign.** This sign is positive if the percussion elicits a contraction of the facial muscles and upper lip. The Chvostek sign is normal in newborns and does not indicate hypocalcemia. If you find a positive Chvostek sign in an adult accompanied by other signs and symptoms such as fatigue, weakness, numbness, or tingling of hands, feet, and facial muscles, a **Trousseau test** must be performed. This test is performed by inflating the blood pressure cuff on the arm to a pressure higher than the patient's systolic blood pressure and looking for the presence of carpal spasm (i.e., flexion of the metacarpophalangeal joint with extension of the interphalangeal joints). If you find this, the Trousseau sign is positive.

CN VIII: Acoustic Nerve

This cranial nerve has two principal functions: **hearing** (cochlear division) and **equilibrium** (vestibular function).

HEARING ASSESSMENT   Hearing requires an intact anatomy of the neural pathway from the cochlea to the inferior colliculus to the cerebral cortex as well as an intact conduction system of the middle ear. Perform a **quick acuity test** by occluding the tragus and testing the capacity to hear a whispered sound (normally it is possible to hear at least 0.7–1.0 m away) and a wristwatch sound (possible to hear at 0.75 m) or a sound made by rubbing the fingers together. If you detect a hearing loss, you will have to discern if the problem is due to a *neurosensorial* or *conductive* abnormality. The peripheral anatomy of the ear can be damaged by drugs such as aspirin, aminoglycosides, and diuretics (e.g., furosemide). The conductive system can be affected by degenerative changes such as otosclerosis. Hearing is assessed by using a tuning fork of 256 Hertz. Review the following tests.

Weber test. Place the vibrating tuning fork over the middle of the vertex of the skull or on the forehead. Then ask the patient whether the sound is heard equally on each side or if it is louder on one side than the other. The sound is normally perceived equally in both ears.

In conduction loss, the sound is heard louder in the blocked ear (*lateralization*).
In sensorial loss, the lateralization occurs to the good ear. The affected ear perceives the vibrations less than does the healthy ear.

Rinne test. Place the vibrating fork on the mastoid process until the patient can no longer hear the sound. Then hold it adjacent to the pinnae. The sound can normally be heard longer through the air than through the bone. This indicates a positive Rinne test, which is normal.

In conduction loss, the bone conduction stimuli appears to be louder than the air conduction stimuli.

TABLE 5-4. Diverse Localization and Etiology of Facial Nerve Lesions

Lesions Above the Nuclei			Lesions Below the Nuclei	
Cortical Lesions	Corticospinal Tract Lesions	Nuclear Lesions	Internal Auditory Meatus (IAM) Lesions	Facial Cranial Lesions
Most patients present with paralysis in the inferior half of the face. It can b caused by cortical lesions on the other side. These lesions are accompanied by weakness of the upper arm (UMN).	Lesions occur in any area between the cortex and facial nerve nucleus.	Lesion affects the facial nuclear nuclei. Other brain stem structures would be affected (lemniscus medialis CN V, VN V1 and CN VII nuclei)	Facial nerve enters IAM with CN VIII and pars inter-media nerve within the cavity lies with CN V and CN VI. Lesions are accompanied with diminished form-ation of tears in the eye, tinnitus, vertigo and deaf-ness. Diminished taste over 2/3 of the tongue and hyperacusias.	At this level only will be affected the CN VII and chorda tympani.
Etiology				
Infarcts	Infarct	Tumors	Trauma	Middle ear infections
Trauma	Tumors	Multiple sclerosis	Mastoiditis	Skull fractures
Tumors	Multiple sclerosis	Infarcts	Herpes zoster	Sarcoidosis (lateral affection)
	Amyotrophic lateral sclerosis	Poliomyelitis	Tumors	Guillain-Barré
				Thiamine deficiency
				Lead intoxication
				Bell Palsy (most common)

General Diagnostic Workup Plan

1. MRI/CT Head
2. EMG
3. CBC
4. Electrolytes
5. Vitamin B$_{12}$ levels

CBC = complete blood count; CN = cranial nerve; CT = computed tomography; EMG = electromyography; MRI = magnetic resonance imaging; UMN = upper motor neuron.

In sensorial loss, both air and bone conduction are diminished, but the air conduction lasts longer than the bone conduction.

Hearing loss is a common complaint that the general practitioner encounters in clinical practice, especially in elderly patients. It is important to ask the patient about the time of presentation and progression of symptoms. The practitioner should also ask if it is a chronic, progressive, or acute problem; if there is a relationship to a particular event (trauma, noise exposure); what medications the patient uses (ototoxics, furosemide, aminoglycosides); if there is a family history of hearing loss; and the pres-

TABLE 5–5. Differential Diagnosis of Bell Palsy

Characteristics	Differential Diagnosis	Diagnostic Workup Plan
Most common form of facial paralysis	1. Tumors of the temporal bone (carotid body, cholesteatoma)	1. EMG
Lower motor neuron (LMN) lesion	2. Ramsay Hunt syndrome*	2. CBC
Incidence is 23 per 100,000 yearly	3. Acoustic neuromas	3. Head CT/MRI
Pathogenesis and etiology unknown; may be hereditary factor and viral etiology	4. Infarcts	4. Electrolytes
Onset is abrupt, unilateral, maximal weakness is attained by 48 hours	5. Guillain—Barré syndrome	
Loss of taste sensation unilaterally and hyperacusis exist		
Pain behind the ear may precede the paralysis for a day or two		
Many patients relate this disorder to exposure to cold weather		

CBC = complete blood count; CT = computed tomography; EMG = electromyogram; MRI = magnetic resonance imaging.
*Due to herpes zoster infection. Severe facial palsy associated with vesicular eruption in the pharynx and external auditory canal.

ence (seen in *acoustic neurinoma*) or absence of vertigo. Table 5–6 lists the differential diagnosis for hearing loss.

OTOSCOPY   Have the SP sit down, and then hyperextend his or her head approximately 30°. Grasp the auricle firmly (but softly), pulling it upward, back, and slightly out; for children, only pull the auricle back. Insert the largest speculum that the ear canal will accommodate. Then observe the ear canals, the tympanic membrane, and note any abnormalities (see Figure 3–3).

VESTIBULAR FUNCTION   The vestibular component of CN VIII perceives acceleration and deceleration movement as well as static perception of the body and its parts in space. **Vertigo** is the cardinal symptom of vestibular disease. Vertigo can be referred to a feeling of spinning, tumbling, and an earthquake-like sensation. It must be differentiated from imbalance, lightheadedness, and syncope, all of which are usually of nonvestibular origin. Vertigo can be accompanied by nausea and vomiting. The physical exam of a patient with vertigo may include the following:

Romberg test. See the Coordination section of this chapter.
Gait observation. See the Motor System Examination section of this chapter.
Fukuda test. Ask the patient to walk with the eyes closed. Always stay close to the patient in case he or she loses balance. The test is considered positive when the patient rotates, usually toward the side of the affected labyrinth.

It is also important to observe if the patient has **nystagmus.** There are several tests that can aid in the diagnosis of positional nystagmus but they are of limited use, especially when the patient is able to fixate. In peripheral lesions, nystagmus tends to be rotatory. In central lesions nystagmus tends to be vertical and develops gradually. Fur-

TABLE 5–6. Differential Diagnosis of Hearing Loss

Conductive Hearing Loss	Sensorial Hearing Loss
Otitis externa	Medications
Cerumen impaction	Aging
Foreign body	Infection (meningitis sequelae)
Tympanosclerosis	Vascular events
Tympanic perforation	Trauma
Stenosis and neoplasms of the canal	Tumor (acoustic neurinoma)*
	Ménière disease

General Diagnostic Workup Plan
1. Audiometry†
2. Speech audiometry‡
3. Tympanometry§
4. CT head scan/MRI
5. MRI

CT = computed tomography; MRI = magnetic resonance imaging.

*These tumors are also called neuromas, or neurilemmomas. All are considered schwannomas because they arise from Schwann cells.

†This study permits the presentation of specific frequencies at specific intensities to each ear by either air or bone conduction. The result of this study is an audiogram (plot of intensity in decibels necessary to reach threshold versus frequency).

‡This study permits the patient to recognize the speech at specific intensity (umbral intensity) as a meaningful symbol.

§This study measures the impedence of sound to the middle ear.

Not every diagnostic test is necessary. Use your own criteria case by case.

thermore, it is possible to have a vestibular affection without vestibular symptoms, as in the case of acoustic neurinoma. Table 5–7 lists the differential diagnosis for vertigo. One important test is the **Hallpike maneuver,** which is diagnostic for **benign positional vertigo.** Perform this maneuver by sitting the patient at bedside and then quickly moving the patient from the sitting position to recumbency, with the head tilted 30° over the end of the table and 30° to one side.

Tests used to evaluate vestibular function are seldom included in a routine neurologic examination. If you consider performing vestibular function tests, you can order them in the diagnostic workup plan of the medical note (see Table 5–7). If you need more information about this topic, consult neurology or otolaryngology textbooks.

CN IX and CN X: Glossopharyngeal and Vagus Nerves

These nerves are tested together because both are affected frequently. Both nerves provide the motor and sensitive innervation to the soft palate and pharynx. CN IX gives innervation for salivation and taste to the posterior one-third of the tongue. CN X provides sensation and motor innervation to the larynx as well as parasympathetic innervation of the thoracic and abdominal organs. To examine these nerves, pay special attention to any hoarseness or nasal quality in the patient's speech. Then tell the patient to open his or her mouth, to say "ah" or to yawn, and observe the soft palate and uvula motion (palate moves upward and uvula inward). The movement must be symmetric. Inspect for any asymmetry. Finally, while warning the patient first and then using a tongue depressor, test the **gag reflex** and inspect for any asymmetry on the palate movement—normal is symmetric (glossopharyngeal exam).

A single lesion of the IX nerve is very rare but can be seen in **glossopharyngeal**

TABLE 5–7. Differential Diagnosis of Vertigo

Acute Vestibular Neuronitis	Benign Positional Vertigo	Ménière Disease	Central Vertigo
Often diagnosed in patients with a history of acute vertigo, commonly with vomiting, ataxia, and malaise	A more specific, peripheral vestibular dysfunction Vertigo attacks are typically triggered by lying down in bed on one side Head movements also exacerbate vertigo	Characterized by paroxysms of vertigo that occur accompanied by persistent unilateral tinnitus Due to distension of the endolymphatic space May be accompanied by hearing loss (low frequency) Well-known causes include syphilis and head trauma	Persists longer than peripheral vertigo and is postural-related More likely to be delayed in onset or due to fatigue after posture change than benign positional vertigo Causes include brain stem vascular disease, A-V malformations, brain stem tumors, and multiple sclerosis

General Diagnostic Workup

1. Caloric stimulation tests
2. CT head scans
3. Audiologic evaluation
4. Electronystagmography (objective recording of nystagmus)
5. Brain stem auditory evoked potential studies
6. MHATP/FTA-ABS

A-V = arteriovenous; CT = computed tomography; MHATP/FTA-ABS = microhemagglutination assay for antibodies to *Treponema pallidum.*

neuralgia, which is characterized by having paroxysms of pain in the tongue, soft palate, or tonsil and are triggered by chewing, swallowing, protruding the tongue, or simply yawning. Single lesions of the vagus nerve (CN X pair) are more common. Paralysis of the recurrent laryngeal nerve (vagus branch, manifested by hoarseness) can be related to a malignant invasion of the mediastinal nodes of the left side (left side lesions are more common due to anatomy), an aortic aneurysm, or after thyroid surgery. If lesions of these nerves are peripheral, the sensitivity of the palate and pharynx as well as the gag reflex can be diminished. In central lesions it is less probable to have decreased sensation, but there is frequently a hyperactive reflex. This is a manifestation of pseudobulbar palsy. Other causes that affect these nerves can be Arnold-Chiari malformation, poliomyelitis, and lateral medullary infarction.

CN XI: Spinal Accessory Nerve

This is motor nerve of the sternocleidomastoid and the superior half of the trapezius muscles. Initially examine these muscles by inspecting the presence of fasciculations or atrophy. Ask the patient to elevate his or her shoulder initially without resistance, then with resistance (upward against your hands). Note any abnormality in strength. Clinical alterations include hemiplegia that can present a delay in shoulder shrug.

CN XII: Hypoglossal Nerve

This nerve innervates the tongue. You can assess this nerve while you are examining CN IX and X. Observe the tongue and look for asymmetry and fasciculations. Then ask the patient to move his or her tongue from side to side and note any abnormality of the movements. Unilateral lesions of the upper motor neuron have little effect on tongue function, although it may present a slight deviation to the side of the lesion. With unilateral lower motor lesions, the tongue deviates to the paralyzed side and atrophy and fasciculations develop. Bilateral involvement of the lower motor neuron is related to a bulbar palsy.

MOTOR SYSTEM EXAMINATION

In addition to the MSE, you can perform a simple screening test if the patient does not have a neurologic problem. During the test try to discern the following:

Localized hemiparesis. Disease from above the magnum foramen.
Segmental disease. Medullary or root nerve disease.
Peripheral disease. Mononeuropathy or polyneuropathy.

To examine the motor system proceed in the following order: **inspection, muscle tone exam, muscle strength exam,** and **coordination.** These tests and the sensory tests can be performed from head to feet, always comparing each side.

Inspection

It is important to observe the patient when he or she follows several commands. Note any abnormalities that occur while the patient is following the command. Always stay close to the patient because of the risk of falling.

Walking. Ask the patient to walk across the room forward and backward. Pay special attention to any abnormality in posture, balance, or gait.
Heel-to-toe test. Then ask the patient to walk heel-to-toe in a straight line, first on the toes and then on the heels. Look for weakness or ataxia.

Finally, inspect in a general manner any obvious problems, such as atrophy, fasciculations, or other abnormal movements. Examine the big group of muscles on the limbs, shoulder, and back as well as the small muscles of the thenar and hypothenar eminencies, searching for the above abnormalities.

Muscle Tone Examination

This consists of several tests that evaluate muscle resistance to passive stretch throughout the body. In general, you can perform these tests by taking one extremity, performing an extension and flexion movement, and measuring the resistance. **Spasticity** is the resistance to passive stretch. Any intent of participation by the patient in the movement of the extremity does not mean increased muscular tone, but it does mean incapacity of relaxation. Muscle tone is diminished in some problems of the corpus callosum, some lower motor neurons, and peripheral nerves; in cerebellar diseases, and in myopathic problems. Muscle tone is increased in the majority of basal ganglia and upper and lower motor neuron lesions (Table 5–8). During passive movements of joints, also test for **rigidity, clonus,** and **hypotonus.** Perform the following examinations:

Move the shoulders to try to determine range of motion
Flexion and extension of the elbow
Flexion and extension of the wrist
Flexion and extension of the fingers
Pronation and supination of the forearm
Flexion and extension at the knee
Flexion and extension of the ankle

Muscle Strength Examination

First, ask the patient about his or her dominant side. You can write this information in your notes. The dominant side is usually stronger. The general form of testing muscle

TABLE 5–8. Upper and Lower Motor Lesions

Upper Motor Lesions	Lower Motor Lesions
Muscle weakness	Muscle weakness
Increased deep tendon reflexes	Depressed deep tendon reflexes
An extensor plantar response (Babinski and Hoffmann signs)*	Fasciculations present
	Important atrophy
No fasciculations	Flaccidity
Mild atrophy	Absent abdominal responses
Spasticity	
Absent abdominal responses	

*Babinski sign indicates upper motor neuron disease. It also occurs in unconscious states associated with drug or alcohol intoxication. It is normal during infancy. It can be elicited by stimulating the lateral aspect of the sole from the heel to the ball of the foot, curving medially across the ball using a sharp object (e.g., a key). Hoffmann sign is performed on the superior limb and is less specific than the Babinski sign. It can be elicited by stimulating the middle finger with the hand in dorsiflexion and observing if dorsiflexion of the thumb develops.

strength is by asking the patient to move the body part actively against your resistance or by resisting your movement, against gravity alone or with gravity eliminated. If the patient fails to move the body part, you must pay close attention to detect a weak muscle contraction or no movement. In your notes you will classify muscle power using a notation such as 5/5 or 2/5. This notation is determined using the following scale:

0 = no muscular contraction (total paralysis)
1 = flicker contraction
2 = movement possible with gravity eliminated
3 = movement against gravity only
4 = movement against gravity and with some resistance
5 = normal power

The first step in evaluating muscle strength is asking the patient to stand up with his or her eyes open for 30 seconds, holding the arms straight in front with the palms up at a 90° angle. Check if there is any difficulty in maintaining the arms in that position. No changes are expected in a healthy person, but in patients with hemiparesis a *downward drift* of one arm with flexion of elbows and fingers is expected. In such a case, you need to document it on your notes as right or left *pronator drift positive*. Then continue testing the following group of muscles on the upper limb in the following order and by asking the italicized questions:

Raising arms (Figure 5–8). Ask the patient to raise his or her arms over the head with the palms forward for 30 seconds making a 180° angle. Observe any alteration such as drifting or weakness on either side, which could suggest hemiparesis. *Can you raise your arms for me?*

Shoulder shrug. Observe any asymmetry during this procedure. You can skip this section if you have already checked CN XI. *Can you shrug your shoulders?* (see Figure 5–8)

Depression of extended arms. Try to depress the patient's outstretched arm sideways as he or she makes a 90° angle. If there is no muscle weakness detected, you can apply resistance against the arm and then ask the patient to push against the wall with the extended arm making a 90° angle. Observe any winging, meaning weak anterior serratus muscle (i.e., the description of the skin over the scapula when the inferior tip of it rotates and moves medially). *Can you push against the*

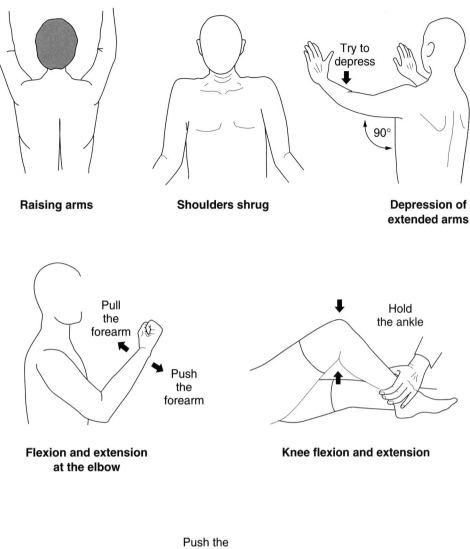

Raising arms   **Shoulders shrug**   **Depression of extended arms**

Try to depress

90°

Pull the forearm

Push the forearm

Hold the ankle

Flexion and extension at the elbow   **Knee flexion and extension**

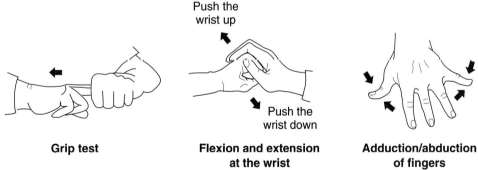

Push the wrist up

Push the wrist down

Grip test   **Flexion and extension at the wrist**   **Adduction/abduction of fingers**

FIGURE 5–8. Muscle strength examination tests.

wall with your extended arm? (At the same time, try to depress the outstretched arm against the SP's resistance; see Figure 5–8.)

Flexion and extension at the elbow. Ask the patient to pull and push his or her forearm against the resistance by your hand. Note the strength by holding the patient's forearm and asking the following questions. Flexion: *Can you pull your forearm to your body?* Extension: *Can you push your forearm toward me?* (see Figure 5–8)

Flexion and extension at the wrist. Ask the patient to resist while you push his or her wrist up or down. Flexion: *Can you pull your hands toward yourself?* Extension: *Can you push your hands toward me?* (see Figure 5–8)

Grip test. Ask the patient to squeeze your fingers. Normally, you will have difficulty in removing your fingers from the patient's grip. Record any weak grip in your notes. *Can your fingers squeeze my fingers?* (see Figure 5–8)

Adduction/abduction of fingers. Test adduction of the fingers by asking the patient to hold your thumb tightly as you pull your thumb between his or her thumb and fingers. To test abduction, ask the patient to try to open his or her fingers in a spread form as you resist the attempt with your hand. *Can you open/close your fingers?* (see Figure 5–8)

Test the muscle strength and assess the extension, flexion, lateral bending, and rotation of the trunk. Respiratory movements can easily be studied as you examine the thoracic cage. In the lower limb, test the flexion and extension of the hip, and so forth:

Flexion and extension of the hip. Ask the patient to raise his or her leg as you try to oppose the movement with your hand over the thigh while the patient is in a supine position or sitting. While the patient is in a prone position, ask him or her to lift the leg. If the patient is standing, ask him or her to kick backward. *Can you lift your leg? Can you kick backward?* (see Figure 3–13)

Adduction/abduction of the hip. Ask the patient to try to spread his or her legs against the force that is being applied (**abduction**). Then put your hands between the knees and ask the patient to close the legs, opposing the force (**adduction**). *Can you open your legs to the side?* (see Figure 3–13)

Knee flexion and extension. With the SP in supine position, flex the knee completely with the patient's foot resting on the bed at approximately 100°. Then put one hand over the knee (anterior side) and hold the ankle with the other hand. Ask the patient to try to straighten the leg as you hold the ankle. Note the force. Repeat the same maneuver by placing one hand under the knee (posterior or popliteal side) and then asking the patient to try to straighten the leg as you resist the movement with your hand over the ankle (extension). Finally, perform the same tests on the contralateral leg. Note all findings. Extension: *Can you kick your foot?* Flexion: *Can you bend your knee?* (see Figure 5–8)

Plantar flexion/dorsiflexion. Ask the patient to push down and pull up against your resistance. Plantar flexion: *Can you step on the brake?* Dorsiflexion: *Can you push against my fingers?*

Symmetrical weakness of the proximal muscles usually suggests myopathy; symmetrical weakness of distal muscles suggests polyneuropathy. When examining any joint movement and muscle strength, always consider associated abnormalities, such as limited range of motion due to articular problems and muscle bulk mass development.

Coordination

Assess coordination by examining the upper and lower limbs as follows:

Romberg test. This test is considered positive when the patient stands with the feet together, the arms and hands not holding onto anything for support, and loses balance—ataxic—when the eyes are closed but not when they are open. This is due to loss of proprioception (decreased position sense). If the patient has **ataxia** or incoordination from cerebellar origin, he or she may have difficulty standing with the feet together with the eyes either open or closed.

Upper limbs. Instruct the patient to perform rapidly alternating movements with his or her hands or arms. The movements can be circling movements with both hands at the same time or with the fingers (e.g., counting numbers with the fingers on both hands simultaneously). Then ask the patient to perform the **finger-nose test:** ask the patient to touch his or her nose first and then touch your finger, which should be held approximately half meter (1.6 ft) from the patient. In

cerebellar ataxia, an intention tremor emerges that is more apparent when the patient approaches the target (your finger). In your notes document the intention tremor as **hypermetria** if the patient reaches beyond the target; record it as **hypometria** if the patient's finger bounces off the target in an uncontrolled fashion. In both cases, the error is corrected by a series of secondary movements as the finger approaches its target, may assume a rhythmic quality, and has traditionally been referred to as **intention tremor.**

Lower limbs. The lower limbs are assessed by the **heel-knee-shin test.** Ask the patient to tap your hand with his or her foot. Note any slowness or tremor during these tests that may be related to cerebellar diseases. In cerebellar diseases the movements tend to be slow, jerky, and clumsy. Rhythmic movements and gross sensory loss are also impaired in extrapyramidal disease.

SENSORY EXAM

Examination of the sensory system is difficult and often fatigues the patient. It also depends on the patient's subjective responses, which may not be accurate. The sensory exam starts with the medical history. The validity of the patient's information is very important, because the patient needs to participate and interpret, in conjunction with the clinician, what he or she feels during the neurologic evaluation. The initial approach consists of a test to evaluate **general sensory functions,** such as pain, temperature, position, and vibration. If the patient is confident and the clinical history suggests a thoughtful clinical exam, then you can examine more **complex sensitive functions,** such as stereognosis and extinction.

Start by asking the patient if he or she has a reduced cutaneous sensation, numbness, or tingling. Then localize the anatomic area where the patient has the alteration of sensation and test it. It is important that you be familiar with the normal dermatome distribution, especially in the upper and lower limbs (see Figure 5–3). As with any other part of the neurologic system, you should perform the assessment as your own clinical criteria dictate.

Perform the sensitivity test in a symmetric manner. For example, if you test the right arm, compare it with the left arm. In real practice, sterilized needles or disposable purpose sharps are used to test pain or two-point discrimination, a wisp of cotton to test light touch, and a 128-Hz tuning fork to test vibration. If you detect an area with sensory loss or hyposensitivity, map the area and indicate if dermatomes are involved (sensation may not be dermatomal) in your notes. Test sensation on the arms, trunk, and legs. The sensory exam is performed with the patient's eyes closed. These tests are divided as follows.

General Sensory Functions

General sensory functions are evaluated using the following tests:

Light touch. Using a wisp of cotton, touch different parts of the patient's body symmetrically and bilaterally. Ask the patient how it feels comparatively. Cotton is provided in the CSA exam rooms.

Pain. You can use the toothpicks provided to you in the CSA exam rooms as a point stimulus. You can use different parts (*blunt* or *pointed* parts) of any other object (e.g., a key) to stimulate the patient's body and then ask the patient if he or she feels a *sharp* or *dull* sensation and generally how the object feels. Pain is increased in radicular diseases and on occasion in polyneuropathy diseases. In these cases, it can be referred to as frank pain, hyperalgesia, or hyperesthesia. As mentioned, tooth picks are used instead of pins on the CSA exam and are provided in the exam rooms.

Temperature. This test is normally omitted. If you need to perform this test, use a few test tubes filled with cold and hot water. Then ask the patient to identify which one is cold and which one is hot. You probably will not have to perform this test, because you will not have the material during the CSA exam.

Position. Take one finger of the patient's hand between your thumb and index finger. Ask the patient to close his or her eyes. Hold the patient's finger at his side and ask him or her to identify whether you are moving the finger down or up. Repeat the maneuver with the big toe.

Vibration. Using a 128-Hz tuning fork, first test the finger by applying the vibrating base of the fork to the pulp of the finger or in the knuckle of the distal interphalangeal joint. Perform the same maneuver on the big toe. Then ask the patient what he or she feels and when the vibrations stop (touch the fork to stop it). If vibration sense is impaired, continue the test on more proximal bony prominences, such as the wrists, elbows, patella, and iliac spines. Vibration sense is often the first sensory function to be lost in peripheral neuropathy. Common causes include diabetes, alcoholism, and aging. Different tuning forks will be available in the CSA exam rooms.

Complex Sensory Functions

The following maneuvers test the cortical ability to correlate, analyze, and interpret sensations. Therefore, these tests are performed if you suspect cortical diseases, especially problems that affect the parietal lobes. In general, parietal lobe lesions cause problems in intellectual processing of sensory (nondominant lesion) and verbal (dominant lesion) information. A lesion in the parietal cortex can impair but not abolish pain, temperature, and sensation to touch. Position sensation is frequently affected but vibration sense is not. Evaluate these functions by performing the following tests while the SP's eyes are closed:

Stereognosis is the ability of the SP, while his or her eyes are closed, to identify objects in the hand. Place a familiar object in the patient's hand (pencil, clip, cotton ball) and ask him or her to identify it. Loss of this ability is called astereognosis. It occurs in posterior column and cortical lesions, respectively.

Two-point discrimination. Use two toothpicks or a specially designed compass graded in centimeters. A healthy, young adult can detect a separation of 3 mm on the finger tips, 1 cm on the palm of the hand, and 3 cm on the sole of the foot. Compare with analogous sites on the two sides of the body. Loss of this ability occurs in posterior column lesions as well as in cortical lesions.

Graphesthesia. Using a blunt-end object such as a pencil or opened paper clip, draw a letter or number on the patient's palm. A patient should normally be able to recognize what is drawn.

Touch localization. Briefly touch the patient's skin anywhere, then ask him or her to open the eyes and point out the place that was touched. Normally a person can recognize the place accurately.

Extinction. Stimulate both sides of the body simultaneously. Ask the patient to tell you where the touch was felt. A healthy person can feel both stimuli. If a cortical lesion exists, only one stimuli will be recognized. The stimulus on the opposite side of the damaged cortex is extinguished.

Loss of position and vibration senses suggests *posterior column disease*. Loss of position and vibration senses but intact light touch and two-point discrimination can be due to *tabes dorsalis, medullar epidural tumors*, or *cervical spondylosis*. Symmetric sensory loss suggests *polyneuropathy*. These losses will be accompanied by decreased deep tendon reflexes (DTRs) as well as decreased appreciation of vibration and position. History of diabetes, alcoholism, or other metabolic disorders supports the diagnosis. Some SPs with a somatoform disorder (e.g., conversion disorder) can have total loss of sensibility in one side of the body. When dealing with such patients, place the tuning fork on one side of the forehead and then on the other. If an organic disease exists, the vibrations will be felt on both sides (due to the fact that the frontal bone is a single structure). Patients with conversion disorder will state that they do not feel the vibrations on one side of the forehead; never confront these patients.

REFLEXES

A reflex is an involuntary response that occurs in response to an external or internal stimulus. The neuron is the structural unit of the nervous system, and the reflex arc is the functional unit. When testing a reflex, you need to note the **speed, force,** and **amplitude of the response.** Always compare one side to the other. If the patient's reflexes are symmetrically diminished or absent, you can use reinforcement. This technique consists of creating an isometric contraction on other muscles that can increase the reflex activity. Before examining the reflexes, the following are examples of reinforcement that can be applied: instruct the patient to clench his or her teeth, squeeze his or her thighs with opposite hands, and hook flexed fingers of two hands together and then attempt to pull them apart (Jendrassik maneuver; Figure 5–9).

Each reflex is graded according to the strength of response as described below:

0 = Absent
1 = Present but diminished. If you use reinforcement, indicate this in your notes.
2 = Just present (average normal)
3 = Brisker than average, may indicate disease
4 = Exaggerated response (hyperactive); often associated with clonus.

Clonus refers to repetitive rhythmic contractions evoked by stretch stimulus. It is most commonly noted at the Achilles tendon. Hyperactive reflexes suggest upper motor neuron disease. Reflexes can be diminished or absent when sensation is lost, when the relevant spinal segments are damaged, or when the lower motor neurons are affected. Neuromuscular diseases also decrease the intensity of a reflex. Document all reflex responses in your notes by using a fraction on a scale (e.g., DTRs 2/4 in lower extremities = normal) or by drawing a human figure as indicated in Figure 5–10. The reflexes marked with an asterisk (*) are the most commonly tested reflexes that can be evaluated during the CSA exam. Review the following groups of commonly performed reflexes.

Upper Limb Reflexes

BICEPS REFLEX (C5–C6)* Place your thumb on the biceps tendon and then strike it with the reflex hammer. Note a flexion at the elbow and be prepared to feel the contraction of the biceps muscle. If there is no response, ask the patient to perform a reinforcement maneuver.

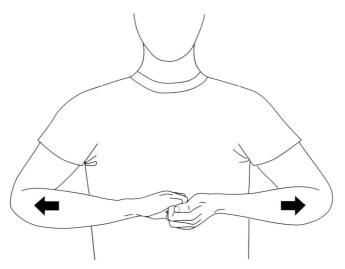

FIGURE 5–9. Jendrassik maneuver.

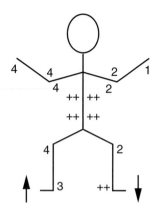

FIGURE 5–10. In the normal adult, the toe plantar flexion are *downgoing*. In upper motor neuron disease (pyramidal lesion), the great toe dorsiflexes (extensor response) with fanning movement of the other toes (Babinski response). Findings would be documented as follows: plantar flexion (normal) = ↓ or downgoing; plantar extension = dorsiflexion, Babinski response = ↑ or upgoing; equivocal = ↑↓. Reflexes are commonly graded from 0 to 4; an average normal response is 2. When recording the figure for muscle stretch reflexes, you can use the + symbols to give a numeric reference for a particular response. A brisker than average response will be 3 (or +++).

TRICEPS REFLEX (C6–C7)*   This test can be performed while the patient is sitting or lying in bed. Flex the patient's arm and the elbow at a 90° angle. Then, holding the arm in this position, strike the triceps tendon above the elbow. Note any contraction of the triceps muscle and extension of the elbow.

SUPINATOR REFLEX (C5–C6)*   With the patient's forearm in a semipronator position, strike the radial border (with the *flat end* of the reflex hammer) of the forearm 3–4 cm above the wrist. Another way to elicit this reflex is by placing your forefinger (index finger) over the tendon and striking over your finger. You will detect a small contraction of the brachioradialis and biceps manifested by a flexion and supination of the forearm.

Lower Limb Reflexes

KNEE REFLEX (L2-L3-L4)*   Perform this test while the patient is sitting with the knees flexed and then relaxed. With the reflex hammer's pointed end, strike the patellar tendon and expect an extension of the knee.

ANKLE REFLEX (S1–S2)*   With the patient relaxed and the knees flexed, hold and slightly dorsiflex the ankle. Then strike the Achilles tendon. In a supine position, you can cross one leg to the other side and have the Achilles tendon exposed to be struck with the hammer. Note the plantar flexion at the ankle and the speed of relaxation after the reflex response.

PLANTAR RESPONSE REFLEX (L4-L5-S1-S2)*   This reflex can be elicited by stimulating the lateral aspect of the sole from the heel to the ball of the foot, curving medially across the ball using a sharp object, such as a key. It is important to hold the ankle firmly, because some patients withdraw the entire leg when the sole is stimulated. After performing the stimulus, note the movement of the toe. **Flexion** is normally expected (*downgoing*, commonly represented as ↓). **Dorsiflexion** (*plantar extension* or *upgoing*, commonly represented as ↑) of the big toe with fanning movement of the other toes constitutes the **Babinski sign** and indicates upper motor neuron (UMN) disease. However, it is normal during infancy. Too intense and uncomfortable a stimulus will lead to withdrawal response. Tables 5–8 and 5–9 list some characteristics of upper motor neuron diseases, lower motor neuron diseases, and clinical examples.

Other Important Reflexes

ABDOMINAL REFLEX*   Using a sharp object, stimulate the abdominal reflex by drawing a line over the abdominal wall across the four segments of the abdomen (see Figure 2–1). Note the contraction of the abdominal muscles and movement of the umbilicus. Abdominal skin muscle reflexes are found in the upper quadrants (T8–T9) and lower quadrants (T11–T12). Perform the umbilical migration test (Beevor sign) if a thoracic lesion is suspected. Lesions at the T9–T10 paralyze the lower abdominal muscles (but maintains intact upper abdominal muscles), resulting in upward movement of the umbilicus (umbilical migration test) when the abdominal wall contracts (Beevor sign).

Cremasteric Reflex (L1–L2)   This test is performed by stimulating the upper inner aspect of the thigh. It normally leads to a retraction of the ipsilateral testicle. (You are not allowed to perform this test during the CSA exam.)

Anal Reflex (S4–S5)   The test is performed by stimulating the skin of the anal margin. There is normally a brisk contraction of the anal sphincter. (You are not allowed to perform this test during the CSA exam under any circumstances. If you consider it pertinent, you can order it on the diagnostic workup plan on the medical note.)

Meningeal Tests

Meningeal tests are not part of the routine neurologic examination. They need to be performed if the medical history suggests the possibility of meningeal irritation (meningitis, subarachnoid hemorrhage). Table 5–10 shows the etiologic agents of meningitis and laboratory tests necessary for diagnosis. Table 5–11 shows bacterial etiologic agents and their frequency by age. Meningeal tests are as follows:

1. **Kernig test.** With the patient in the supine position, flex the hip at a 90° angle with the knee totally flexed (see Chapter 3) and then extend the knee. Resistance or pain during flexion constitutes a positive Kernig sign (Figure 5–11).
2. **Brudzinski test.** With the patient in the supine position, flex the patient's neck forward. Look for flexion of the hips and knees in response to the maneuver or stiffness of the neck. If one of these occurs, it constitutes a positive Brudzinski sign (see Figure 5–11).

TABLE 5–9. Upper and Lower Motor Neuron, Neuromuscular, and Muscle Disease

Upper Motor Neuron Disease	Lower Motor Neuron Disease	Neuromuscular Disease	Muscle Disease
Cerebrovascular disease	Motor neuron disease*	Myasthenia gravis	Duchenne muscular dystrophy
Head or spinal injury	Spinal root disorder	Myasthenic syndrome†	Metabolic myopathies
Tumors	Peripheral nerve disorders		Congenital myopathies
Myotonic disorders			Polymyositis
Diagnostic Workup			
1. CT scan of the head	1. EMG studies	1. Edrophonium test	1. Muscle biopsy
2. CBC (PTLs)	2. CT/MRI	2. EMG studies	2. CK
3. PT, PTT	3. Muscle biopsy	3. Serum assay of antiacetylcholine antibodies	3. ESR
4. LFTs	4. Myelography		4. Electrolytes
5. BUN/Cr	5. CK	4. Chest radiographs	5. Antinuclear antibodies
		5. CT scan of the thorax	

BUN = blood urea nitrogen; CBC = complete blood count; CK = creatine kinase; Cr = creatinine; CT = computed tomography; EMG = electromyogram; ESR = erythrocyte sedimentation rate; LFT = liver function tests; PT = prothrombin time; PTLs = platelets; PTT = partial thromboplastin time.

*Amyotrophic lateral sclerosis (ALS) is the most common form of progressive motor neuron disease.

†Eaton Lambert syndrome, or myasthenia-like syndrome, is seen in association with bronchogenic carcinoma. This syndrome is characterized by weakness, myalgias, and fatigability, often most severe in the lower extremities and proximal muscles. In these patients, the diagnostic workup also will include chest radiographs, sputum cytology, and bronchoscopy.

TABLE 5–10. Meningitis

Clinical Manifestations	Classification	Etiology	Differential Diagnosis	Diagnostic Workup Plan
Headache	Bacterial	**Bacterial**	1. Brain abscess	1. LP → CSF examination
Fever	Aseptic (viral)	**(see Table 5-11)**	2. Subarachnoid hemorrhage	2. CT head scan
Positive Brudzinski and Kernig signs	Chronic or recurrent	**Viral**	3. Encephalitis	3. VDRL
Nausea, vomiting		Enteroviruses	4. CNS neoplasms	4. ELISA (IgM, IgG antibodies)
Profuse sweating, weakness		Arboviruses	5. CNS syphilis	
		HIV	6. Lyme disease (neurologic symptoms)	5. CBC, Electrolytes
Myalgias, photophobia		HSV-2		
		Chronic or Recurrent		
		Candida albicans		
		Nocardia asteroides		
		Histoplasma capsulatum		
		Mycobacterium tuberculosis		
		Actinomyces israelii		

CBC = complete blood count; CNS = central nervous system; CSF = cerebrospinal fluid; ELISA = enzyme linked immunosorbent assay; HIV = human immunodeficiency virus; HSV = herpes simplex virus; IgG = immunoglobulin G; IgM = immunoglobulin M; LP = lumbar puncture; VDRL = Venereal Disease Research Laboratory.
*Not every test is necessary. Use your own criteria case by case.

WRITING NOTES FOR A NEUROLOGIC EXAM

The following section contains samples of written notes for a neurologic exam. Review the complete and abbreviated forms.

Neurologic Exam *(Detailed format of a patient with chronic inflammatory demyelinating polyneuropathy) (Extended format)*

Speech is fluent and coherent. This is a R. handed patient and he is alert and oriented in space, time, and person. Mini-mental status examination is 30/30. Cranial nerves II-XII are grossly within normal limits. His gait had a slightly wide base and is waddling. Motor examination of the upper extremities showed strength of 5/5 in both the proximal and distal muscles. In the lower extremities the left proximal muscles showed a strength of 4/5, and in the distal muscles

TABLE 5–11. Bacterial Etiologic Agents of Meningitis by Age

Patient Age	Bacterial CNS Infections (Etiologic Agent)
Children younger than 1 month	Enteric gram negative; *Escherichia coli* (70%), *Listeria monocytogenes*
Children older than 1 month	*Haemophilus influenzae* (60%) *Neisseria meningitides* (20%) *Streptococcus pneumoniae* (20%)
Children with shunt insertions	*Staphylococcus epidermidis* (92%–99%) *Staphylococcus aureus* (1%–8%)
Patients older than 15 years	*S. pneumoniae* (30%–50%) *N. meningitides* (10%–35%) Staphylococci (5%–15%)

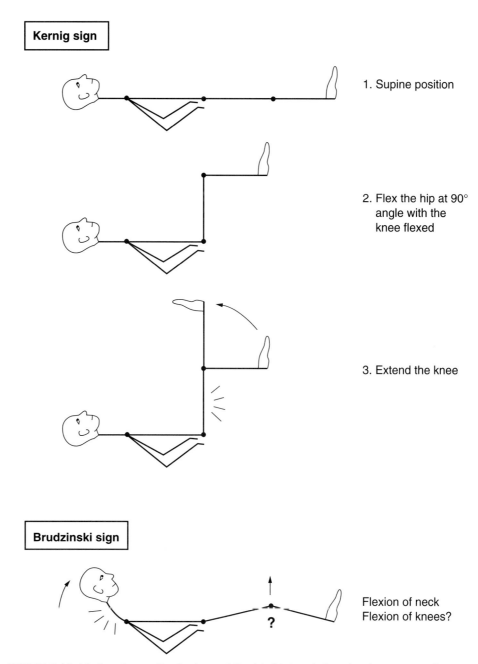

Kernig sign

1. Supine position

2. Flex the hip at 90°
   angle with the
   knee flexed

3. Extend the knee

Brudzinski sign

Flexion of neck
Flexion of knees?

?

FIGURE 5–11. Meningeal tests: Kernig sign and Brudzinski sign. (Adapted with permission from Pryse-Philips W, Murray TJ: *Essential Neurology,* 2nd ed. Garden City, New York: Medical Examination Publishing Company, 1982. Spanish edition.)

the patient had 0/5 (both plantar flexion and ankle plantar flexion were also 0/5). On the right side, the patient had proximal muscle strength of 4+/5, and in the distal muscles the patient had 1/5 ankle dorsiflexion and 4–/5 plantar flexion. There are no fasciculations. The cerebellar examination is limited by his weakness and is grossly within normal limits. The finger-to-nose test did not reveal any dysmetria. The sensory examination showed glove and stocking pattern loss of all the modalities in the lower extremities up to the middle of the thigh and the upper extremities up to the middle of the forearm. The deep tendon reflexes in the upper extremities and lower extremities are 2/4 without any reinforcement, although there is a loss of bilateral ankle jerks. The plantar responses are downgoing.

Neuro (Concise format)

MSE and speech were normal.
CN: II-XII within normal limits.
Motor: L. leg proximal muscles 4/5; distal muscles 0/5.
    R. leg proximal muscles 4+/5; distal m. 1/5, ankle dorsiflexion and plantar flexion 4-/5. Other muscles normal strength, coordination normal.
Coordination: Unremarkable.
Sensitive: Glove and stocking pattern loss to all modalities in both legs.
Reflexes: DTRs 2/4 on both knees, plantar downgoing (both).

Neuro (Relative concise format)

MSE: Lying in bed, somewhat suspicious. Poor grooming. Attentive, guarded. Fair eye contact. Speech normal rate, rhythm, tone, volume and content. Patient is alert and oriented X3.
Cranial nerves: II-X are grossly within normal limits, XI CN exam shows significant sternocleidomastoid and trapezius muscle wasting with power of 2/5, XII CN exam reveals tongue fasciculations, dysarthria, nasal quality, often unintelligible, weakness noted in lingual and gutter muscle.
Motor system: Showed significant weakness in the range of 2–3 in all muscle groups, strongest being the right wrist flexors 3+/5.
Sensory system: Unremarkable.
Reflexes: 2/4 in right upper extremity. Jaw jerk 3/4 fasciculations noted in the left forearm. Cerebellar not tested due to extreme weakness.

Neurological Exam (Concise format)

MMSE: 29/30 (−1 for date) but performed with difficulty.
CN: Mild left facial drop, central type, minimal decrease sensations on V1-V3 on the left side. Other CN are intact.
Motor system: 5/5 on all muscles tested. Gait with cane due to old ankle fracture.
    Coordination was unremarkable.
Sensory system: ↓ sensation in stocking distribution up to the ankle level reflexes; DTR 1/4 symmetrically.

Neurologic (Concise format)

Alert, well oriented X3. Cranial nerves normal. Motor 5/5. Sensory intact to pin, vibration, and proprioception. DTRs were 3/4. Plantar reflexes ↓.

Neuro. Exam (Concise format)

Alert well oriented X3, satisfactorily groomed, appearing stated age. Speech fluent with normal volume and content. II-XII CNs normal. Group by group motor exam revealed ↓ strength (4/5) for the R. wrist and finger flexors. Hypersensitivity to sharp stimulus was detected in the C5, C6 dermatomes and hyposensitivity on the C7 dermatome. DTRs showed 2/4 responses symmetrically.

Neuro *(Concise format)*

MS: Cooperative, well oriented ×3. Speech normal in rate and volume.

CNs: VII CN reveals weakness on the R. side when smiling.

Motor: Gait was limited by R. leg movement, but possible. Positive pronator drift on right arm. Significant muscle weakness of 2/5 on the R. leg and R. arm. Coordination was normal.

Sensory: Decreased sensation to all modalities on the right side of the body.

Reflexes:

6

Psychiatry: Writing Medical Notes

INTRODUCTION

The psychiatric medical history is done following the general format described in Chapter 3. The purpose of the psychiatric history is the same as that of other medical histories: to obtain the history of the present illness (HPI), past medical history (PMH), family history (FH), psychiatric history, and so on, and to address the relationship between events in the patient's life and the current emotional issues (Figure 6–1). In addition, information about neurovegetative symptoms, such as libido, appetite, and sleep, must be obtained. The clinical examination of the **patient's mental status**—that is, an individual's current state of mental functioning—is performed under the **mental status examination.** The format discussed in this chapter will be useful when you approach a psychiatric case, as you will be required to do on the day of the CSA exam.

It is also important to be familiar with the multiaxial system from the *Diagnostic and Statistical Manual of Mental Disorders* (DSM-IV). This system facilitates the comprehensive and systematic evaluation of various mental disorders, general medical conditions, psychosocial problems, environmental problems, and patient's level of functioning (Table 6–1).

A) PSYCHIATRIC HISTORY
1. Chief complaint (CC)
2. History of the present illness (HPI)
3. Psychiatric history
4. Past medical history (PMH)
5. Social history (SH)
6. Family history (FH)
7. Developmental psychiatric history
8. Review of systems (ROS)

B) MENTAL STATUS EXAMINATION (MSE)
1. General aspects
2. Mood and affect (emotions)
3. Speech
4. Perception
5. Thought
6. Cognitive and intellectual functions (Mini-Mental Status Examination [MMSE])
7. Impulse control
8. Judgment and insight

C) DIFFERENTIAL DIAGNOSIS
–Plans for dif. diagnosis (1-5)

D) DIAGNOSTIC WORKUP
–Plans for diagnosis (1-5)

Figure 6–1. The format of a psychiatric history and mental status examination (MSE).

TABLE 6–1. Multiaxial System from the *Diagnostic and Statistical Manual of Mental Disorders* (DSM-IV)

Axis I: Clinical disorders

Axis II: Personality disorders, mental retardation

Axis III: Medical condition

Axis IV: Psychosocial and environmental problems

Axis V: Global assessment of functioning (1–100)

(Reprinted with permission from the American Psychiatric Association: *Diagnostic and Statistical Manual of Mental Disorders,* 4th ed. Washington, DC: American Psychiatric Association, 1994, p. 25.)

The multiaxial system provides a convenient format to organize, communicate, and capture the complexity and heterogeneity of clinical situations. An important aspect of this system is that it promotes biopsychosocial models in clinical, educational, and research settings. Axis V is used by the clinician to evaluate the overall level of functioning. It is useful in planning the management and treatment of a case. The overall functioning assessment on Axis V is done using the Global Assessment of Functioning (GAF) scale (Table 6–2).

Some clinicians do not like to use this system. For CSA purposes, the multiaxial system may or may not be helpful, but we include it here as a reference because it is commonly used in different psychiatric notes in real clinical practice. We include some examples at the end of this chapter that might be helpful to you but will not necessarily reflect a note that you will need to write during the CSA exam. During the CSA exam, you will not have access to the GAF scale.

PSYCHIATRIC HISTORY

Most of the information discussed in this chapter has already been described in Chapter 3. The following sections include only the most important information relevant to psychiatric cases; information about any other previously described topics will not be repeated here.

Chief Complaint (CC)

The chief complaint section follows the same format as that for general medical notes. See the following examples:

Chief Complaint

Mr. Thompson is a 47 yo w. male who is admitted because he says, "I am hearing voices telling me a lot of bad things."

Chief Complaint

Miles Duesterberg is a 40-year-old white man with bipolar disorder who states that he has been having chest pain.

Complaint

Mr. Ferguson is a 34 yo w. male with alcohol dependence who came to the emergency room because of agitation, tremors, confusion and is stating that he is "hearing voices."

History of the Present Illness (HPI)

This section follows the same indications as when writing general medical notes. See the following examples:

TABLE 6–2. Global Assessment of Functioning (GAF) Scale

Code	Description
100–91	**Superior functioning in a wide range of activities, life's problems never seem to get out of hand, is sought out by others because of his or her many positive qualities. No symptoms.**
90–81	**Absent or minimal symptoms** (e.g., mild anxiety before an exam), **good functioning in all areas, interested and involved in a wide range of activities, socially effective, generally satisfied with life, no more than everyday problems or concerns** (e.g., an occasional argument with family members).
80–71	**If symptoms are present, they are transient and expectable reactions to psychosocial stressors** (e.g., difficulty concentrating after family argument); **no more than slight impairment in social, occupational, or school functioning** (e.g., temporarily falling behind in schoolwork).
70–61	**Some mild symptoms** (e.g., depressed mood and mild insomnia) **OR some difficulty in social, occupational, or school functioning** (e.g., occasional truancy, or theft within the household), **but generally functioning pretty well, has some meaningful interpersonal relationships.**
60–51	**Moderate symptoms** (e.g., flat affect and circumstantial speech, occasional panic attacks) **OR moderate difficulty in social, occupational, or school functioning** (e.g., few friends, conflicts with peers or co-workers).
50–41	**Serious symptoms** (e.g., suicidal ideating, severe obsessional rituals, frequent shoplifting) **OR any serious impairment in social, occupational, or school functioning** (e.g., no friends, unable to keep a job).
40–31	**Some impairment in reality testing or communication** (e.g., speech is at times illogical, obscure, or irrelevant) **OR major impairment in several areas, such as work or school, family relations, judgment, thinking, or mood** (e.g., depressed man avoids friends, neglects family, and is unable to work; child frequently beats up younger children, is defiant at home, and is failing at school).
30–21	**Behavior is considerably influenced by delusions or hallucinations OR serious impairment in communication or judgment** (e.g., sometimes incoherent, acts grossly inappropriately, suicidal preoccupation) **OR inability to function in almost all areas** (e.g., stays in bed all day; no job, home, or friends).
20–11	**Some danger of hurting self or others** (e.g., suicide attempts without clear expectation of death; frequently violent; manic excitement) **OR occasionally fails to maintain minimal personal hygiene** (e.g., smears feces) **OR gross impairment in communication** (e.g., largely incoherent or mute).
10–1	**Persistent danger of severely hurting self or others** (e.g., recurrent violence) **OR persistent inability to maintain minimal personal hygiene OR serious suicidal act with clear expectation of death.**
0	Inadequate information.

The rating of overall psychological functioning on a scale of 0–100 was operationalized by Luborsky in the Health-Sickness Rating Scale (Luborsky L: "Clinicians' Judgments of Mental Health." *Archives of General Psychiatry* 7:407–417, 1962). Spitzer and colleagues developed a revision of the Health-Sickness Rating Scale called the Global Assessment Scale (GAS) (Endicott J. Spitzer RL, Fleiss JL, Cohen J: "The Global Assessment Scale: A Procedure for Measuring Overall Severity of Psychiatric Disturbance." *Archives of General Psychiatry* 33:766–771, 1976). A modified version of the GAS was included in DSM-III-R as the Global Assessment of Functioning (GAF) Scale.

(Reprinted with permission from the American Psychiatric Association: *Diagnostic and Statistical Manual of Mental Disorders*, 4th ed. Washington, DC: American Psychiatric Association, 1994, p 32.)

History of the Present Illness (Extended format)

The patient came on his own to be admitted due to a relapse of voices. He has been compliant with his medications, but he has been hearing the voices, telling him to do bad things with no further elaboration. He feels that other people are talking about him, and they are making fun of him as well. He has been feeling more depressed than usual since the voices have started making him feel like this. He feels that no one cares for him. He has been separated from his wife for months. He said that they had been having problems for a long time. He feels that she is quite domineering and controlling. He said that she treats him as if he was a kid and he is a man. He has not been sleeping well, he feels hopeless, with less energy. Many times he walks for miles at a time to relieve the tension he feels.

HPI *(Concise format)*

This previously well pt was admitted on his own due to relapses of hallucinatory voices and a new onset of delusions reported. He has been separated from his wife for months. He describes her as quite domineering and controlling and says that she treats him as if he were a child. He feels depressed and lonely; sometimes he walks for miles trying to relieve his tension.

H. of the Present Illness *(Extended format)*

While being interviewed, the patient reports worsening anxiety and some suicidal thoughts. He denies any suicidal intent and says that he feels in fairly good control of his thoughts. He says he has been upset since yesterday afternoon when he received a phone call from his ex-wife asking him for money and talking about what a good husband he had been. He says that he has accumulated a great deal of credit card debt because he has been giving money to her in order to win her back, and hearing from her brought back all his anger towards her.

Hx P Illness *(Concise format)*

The patient reports worsening anxiety with some suicidal thoughts but no intent. He says he felt well in control of these thoughts. He was well until yesterday evening when he received a call from his ex-wife asking him for money, and hearing from her again brought back all his anger towards her.

HPI *(Concise format)*

Mrs. Brown states that her father (Mr. Barber) had been well until one year ago when he developed memory loss and loss of his intellectual abilities. Initially he started having problems remembering recent events and then he started talking about things that had occurred a long time ago. A month ago he tried to sell one of his properties for a ridiculous price.

HPI *(Concise format)*

This young woman who was seen by me today states that she has a total loss of sensory and motor functions in her left arm. She claims that the symptoms appear suddenly without any precipitant event such as trauma or any relation to a previous illness. She denies dysthesias, fasciculations, or numbness.

Psychiatric History

In the psychiatric history you can include information about neurovegetative symptoms, such as libido, appetite, and sleep. Also include any previous psychiatric problems, medications, and/or relapses of his main current problem as well as the impact of these relapses on the family. You can include this part under PMH, but if you want to be more descriptive you can separate it out as follows:

Psychiatric History

The patient was diagnosed with schizophrenia at the age of 18 while in the Army and treated for 6 months with Thorazine and Stelazine; he was told much later that was a misdiagnosis and started lithium. Patient has also taken Tegretol in the past, which he felt did very little to improve his mood swings.

Psychiatric Hx

Panic disorder was diagnosed 3 years ago, currently on treatment with Imipramine BID. She felt that the Imipramine didn't help her. Relapses were reported one year ago because the patient admitted failing to take the medication.

Psychiatric Hx

Patient states that he was treated with Fluoxetine 2 years ago for a major depressive disorder. Since then he says he was fine and no recurrences were referred. He states that he has no sleep or appetite problems.

Past Medical History (PMH)

This section follows the same indications as writing general medical notes. If you prefer, you can include the past psychiatric history under this category as well, as in the next example. More PMH examples appear in Chapter 3.

Past Medical History (Extended format)

Psychiatric Hx:
Past psychiatric hx includes history of alcohol dependence treated on multiple occasions with benzodiazepines. However, patient has refused rehabilitation/treatment for it since 1 year ago.
Medical H:
NIDDM diagnosed 10 years and 5 years ago.
HTN diagnosed 5 years ago.
Medications:
Glipizide 2.5 mg QD
Captopril 10 mg QD
Aspirin prn
Allergies: None known

PMH (Concise format)

Phobic disorder diagnosed 3 years ago, treated with systematic desensitization treatments. MI 5 years ago treated with thrombolytic tx at the Memorial Hospital. HTN dx 5 years ago. Current medications include aspirin 325 mg QD + propanolol BID.

Social History (SH)

Approach these notes like other general written notes.

In practice, problems related to alcoholism are seen by the psychiatrist, internist, and generalist. It is important to identify an alcoholic patient if you suspect that he or she has a problem. Alcoholism screening is very important to consider on the psychiatric history, although it doesn't necessarily need to go here; it can be used in other situations, and under different formats, depending on the clinical condition of the patient. Alcoholism is a syndrome that consists of two phases: the problem of drinking (repetitive use of EtOH use to relieve anxiety or emotional conditions) and addiction (i.e., a true addiction). The alcoholic patient may have different clinical conditions, depending on the amount of alcohol and the length of time the patient has been drinking (Table 6–3). A common presentation is the patient complaining of tremors, insomnia, blackouts, depression, and so on. Never judge the patient; do not confront him or her. Ask the appropriate questions in a professional manner. The CAGE questionnaire helps the examiner to screen a patient with a probable alcohol problem (Table 6–4). Finally, do not forget to ask if any other member of the family has or has had an alcoholic problem.

Family History

The family history is done just as described in Chapter 3.

TABLE 6–3. Alcohol Abuse and Psychiatric Disorders

Acute Intoxication	Withdrawal	Alcoholic Hallucinosis	Chronic Alcoholic Brain Syndrome
Like any other CNS depressant Drowsiness, Psychomotor dysfunction, dysarthria, ataxia, nystagmus Nausea, vomiting Blood levels < 50 mg rarely cause marked dysfunction. Blood levels >150 mg cause ataxia, dysarthria, nausea, vomiting. Blood levels between 350–900 mg are lethal.	A wide spectrum of anxiety, decreased cognition, tremulousness due to increased irritability and hyperactivity **Delirium tremens** Acute organic psychosis that occurs 25–72 hrs after the last drink. The signs and symptoms include tremors, sensory hyperacuity, visual hallucinations (snakes, bugs). Autonomic hyperactivity, diaphoresis, dehydration and electrolyte disturbances ($K^+\downarrow$, $Mg^+\downarrow$), seizures and cardiovascular abnormalities.	Occurs during heavy drinking or withdrawal. Signs and symptoms consist of paranoid psychosis without tremulousness, confusion and clouded sensorium. Patient can be normal except for auditory hallucinations, delusions of persecution, etc. Patient can be aggressive or paranoid	Encephalopathy characterized by increased erratic behavior, memory and recall problems, and emotional instability. **Wernicke encephalopathy** Due to thiamine deficiency. Is an acute reversible state characterized by ataxia, confusion, nystagmus, and ophthalmoplegia (CN VI paralysis) **Korsakoff psychosis** Due to thiamine deficiency. A chronic, usually irreversible condition characterized by anterograde and retrograde amnesia and confabulation.

Differential Diagnosis

Other CNS depressants such as benzodiazephine or barbiturate overdose	Other sedative withdrawal due to benzodiazepine and other causes of delirium	Other acute paranoid states Amphetamine abuse Psychosis Paranoid schizophrenia	Organic brain syndrome Systemic lupus erythematosus

Diagnostic workup

1. LFTs: ALT, AST, bilirubin total and direct
2. Serum uric acid
3. Triglyceride
4. CBC, MCV
5. Electrolytes (Mg^+)

ALT = alanine aminotransferase; AST = aspartate aminotransferase; CBC = complete blood count; LFTs = liver function tests; MCV = mean cell volume.

TABLE 6–4. CAGE Screening Test*

1. Have you ever felt the need to **cut down** on drinking?
2. Have you ever felt **annoyed** by criticism of your drinking?
3. Have you ever felt **guilty** about your drinking?
4. Have you ever taken a morning **eye opener**†?

*Results: **Two "yes" answers** are considered a positive screen. **One "yes" answer** should arouse suspicion of alcohol abuse.
†This is the term to describe when a patient needs to drink alcohol immediately after awakening.

Developmental Psychiatric History

It is very important to ask about important events that have occurred during the patient's life. Review the following parameters and question list, which can help guide you through the patient's developmental history. Use your own criteria case by case.

Prenatal
Were you a wanted child?
Did your mother have any difficulty during pregnancy and delivery?
Were you discharged from the hospital at the same time as your mother?

Early Childhood (0–3 years)
Earliest recollections? How was your childhood?
Any problems related to feeding, toilet training, sleep?
What was your personality like as a child?
Sibling relationships?

Childhood (3–11 years)
Response to first separation from mother?
Personality patterns (quiet, assertive, aggressive, anxious)?
Development of reading and motor skills?
Peer relationship in school (leader, follower, popular?)
Fears, setting fires, cruelty to animals, nightmares, bed-wetting?

Adolescence
Any emotional problems? (weight, drug use, running away?)
Role models
Relationships with classmates and teachers?
Active in sports?
Sexuality (masturbation, crushes, homosexual behavior, fantasies)

Adulthood
How are your social life and quality of human relationships?
How is your employment history?
Sexual interaction?

(Adapted with permission from Fadem B: *BRS Behavioral Science*, 2e. Philadelphia: Lippincott Williams & Wilkins, 1994, p 132.)

The time that you spend on any particular case will depend on the patient's underlying problem. Use your own criteria in every case; the following examples don't necessarily reflect the number of words that you need to use for the CSA notes.

Developmental History

Childhood and adolescence, states that he was very happy. Patient was raised by grandparents because "mother was a whore" and he was not ever allowed to see her. He states he was spoiled as a child and feels that was a disservice to him as an adult because it has made him irritable. He was always close to his siblings and remains close to his half-sister at this time. No hx of abuse was reported. Level of education: graduated from private high school, some college at Northwestern in Evanston, IL; was accepted at another major university but did not matriculate.

Developmental Hx

No prenatal data were obtained. Early childhood and childhood, states that he was very happy but refers to some sexual interactions described as "touches" with older children. During adolescence he experimented with some homosexual encounters that caused him severe identity conflict. Level of education, graduated from college with master's degree studies, married with two children, his married life is defined as acceptable but refers to still having an identity conflict.

Developmental Hx

Early childhood and childhood, he states that he was very happy. During adolescence he split time between his parents because they divorced when he was 13 years old. At the age of 15 he started using drugs with high school friends; since then he consumes marijuana frequently, up until present. He did not go to college, he is divorced with two children, right now he works in the city as a taxi driver.

Develop. Hx.

Patient's mother states that as a child was quiet, obedient and never formed friendships. The patient states that he dreams of one day knowing the truth about what the pope and church hid from us. He dislikes social activities and never had a girlfriend.

Review of Systems

The review of systems is done in the same manner as explained in Chapter 3.

MENTAL STATUS EXAMINATION (MSE)

The mental status examination and speech evaluation should be done in the context of the interview and the general medical history and physical exam. During the conversation, assess the patient's level of consciousness, and pay special attention to grooming, orientation, personal hygiene, facial expression, mood, affect, speech, and memory. Note the patient's vocabulary in context of his or her culture and level of education: you may be able to make a rough estimate of the patient's intelligence in the course of the interview. The mental status examination is used to describe the clinician's observations and impression of the patient/SP during the interview.

General Aspects of the MSE

Review the following general aspects of the MSE:

Appearance. This includes grooming (e.g., tidy, disheveled), poise, clothing, body type (e.g., childlike), etc. Descriptions can include observations, such as deterioration in grooming and personal hygiene (seen in **depression, schizophrenia, and organic brain syndromes**), excessive fastidiousness (seen in **obsessive-compulsive disorder**), one-sided neglect (in **parietal lesions, nondominant lesion**)

Activity/behavior. This is sometimes called motor or activity; it describes the patient's motor behavior. Document the patient's gait, gestures, coordination, movements, ability to relax, eye contact, immobile parts, changes during the discussion, etc. Describe them as restlessness, tense posture, slumped posture, bizarre posture, tics, expansive movements, etc. Does the patient lie in bed or prefer to walk? Any involuntary movement?

Attitude. This describes the attitude toward the examiner. Note patient's reactions—whether they seem inappropriate, appropriate, or extreme at certain points. Describe as cooperative, guarded, seductive, frank, angry, hostile, etc.

Review the following examples:

General

Appearance: Satisfactorily groomed, appeared stated age
Behavior: Appropriate, good eye contact
Attitude: Cooperative

General

Appearance: Appears stated age, looks overweight
Behavior: Cooperative, decreased activity
Attitude: Appropriate

General

Poorly groomed, markedly restless, stood up and paced around the room several times. He was tremulous, breathing rapidly but in control. At one point he became so agitated that he asked to leave the room, and eventually asked to terminate the interview.

General

Lying in bed, somewhat suspicious, poor grooming, attentive, guarded, fairly good eye contact.

Mood and Affect

Explore how the patient/SP feels and how he expresses his emotional condition. Approach the patient properly and explain your descriptions using the following terminology.

Mood is an internal emotional condition perceived by the patient. In other words, is what the patient says how he feels? You can assess the patient/SP by asking: *How do you feel today? What do you expect for your future? Do you ever feel that life has no sense for you?*

Review the following psychological states:

Euphoria—strong feeling of elation
Expansiveness—feeling of self-importance
Irritability—patient easily bothered and quick to anger
Euthymic—normal mood. No depression, no elevation of mood
Dysphoria—subjective unpleasant feeling
Grief—sadness due to a true loss
Depression—sadness not due to a specific loss
Anhedonia—lack of ability to feel pleasure
Mood swings—Alternations between euphoric and depressive moods

Affect is how the above emotional (mood) conditions are expressed. Document the relationship between the internal emotional condition and its outward expressions. Note if the **affect** is congruent or not.

Review the following psychological states:

Appropriate—congruency between the mood and affect. For example, the patient tells you that he feels euphoric and he looks happy.

Inappropriate—discordance between mood and behavior. For example, a patient tells you that he feels sad due to his recent father's death, but he appears to be very happy.

Restricted affect—reduced display of emotional response

Blunted affect—strongly reduced display of emotional response

Flat affect—lack of emotional response

Labile affect—sudden emotional response not related to the precipitant event. For example, the patient cries easily during the interview when she remembers how she lost her cat 20 years ago.

You can describe **appropriateness,** or how the mood and affect are related. Normally, mood and affect are congruent. In schizophrenia, however, for example, the patient's moods are incongruent. Mood disorders are clinical states characterized by changes in mood due to elevated or diminished mood, both with or without relation to particular events. Particular clinical syndromes vary depending on the clinical state of the patient (e.g., **mania** or **depression**) and the relation of that state to environmental factors, such as life stressor, winter season, postpartum effects, and so on. The different types of mood disorders and their differential diagnoses are listed in Table 6–5.

Finally, one important topic to review is normal grief or bereavement. Grief is a normal reaction characterized initially by shock and denial. The patient/SP normally reports to you that the deceased person is physically present. He or she may avoid social activities, and may feel sad and lonely. Guilt and anger toward the deceased person are an initial reaction. Normal grief usually subsides after 1 to 2 years. The presence of extreme mood disturbances and alteration in sleep patterns might indicate an abnormal reaction. Be explicit and precise in your notes, as in the following examples:

Mood: Depressed
Affect: Sad
Mood: Euthymic
Affect: Appropriate
Mood is euthymic and affect blunted.
Mood irritable, affect congruent, somewhat labile.

Speech

In evaluation of the patient's speech, you should describe the physical characteristics of speech, e.g., **spontaneity, articulation, fluency, quantity, rate and rhythms,**

TABLE 6–5. Mood Disorders

Types of Mood Disorders	Differential Diagnosis*	General Diagnostic Workup Plan
Major depressive disorder	The mood disorders listed, *plus*	Dexamethasone suppression test
Bipolar disorder	Anorexia nervosa	T_3, T_4, TSH
Dysthymic disorder	Anxiety disorders	Electrolytes
Cyclothymic disorder	Schizophrenia	CBC
Seasonal affective disorder	Somatization	
Adjustment disorder with depressed mood	Grief	
Postpartum depression	Drug and alcohol abuse	
	Hypothyroidism	

CBC = complete blood count; T_3 = triiodothyronine; T_4 = thyroxine; TSH = thyroid-stimulating hormone.
*It is not necessary to include every diagnostic possibility in your differential diagnosis. The differential diagnosis may depend on the clinical situation.

volume, and **quality** (appropriate use of words and letters). Note any speech defects, if present, as follows:

Dysarthria—articulation affected without disturbance of language function

Dysphonia—defect of speech volume. Temporary or permanent effect on respiratory muscles or vocal cords

Aphasia—may be an abnormal comprehension aphasia (as from dominant temporal lesions leading to Wernicke aphasia) or poor production of speech (as from dominant lesions on frontal lobes leading to Broca aphasia), or both. Aphasic speech lacks grammatical structure.

Fluency—the amount of speech in a given period of time. Nonfluent speech contains only a limited number of words.

Apraxia—disorder of a skilled movement not attributable to weakness, lack of coordination, or failure in comprehension

Agnosia—the inability to recognize objects that the patient/SP sees, despite intact visual pathways and speech capacity.

For CSA purposes, describe speech in a single note, as in the following examples:

Speech: Fluent and coherent

Speech: Fluent, normal rate and volume. Rapid at times.

Speech: Dysarthric, normal in volume but not in rate.

Perception

Perception refers to the patient's experience in reference to himself and the environment. Describe abnormal perception as follows:

Illusions—misinterpretations of real external stimuli. For example, interpreting the appearance of a coat in dark closet as a man, or hearing rustling leaves as the sound of voices.

Hallucinations—subjective, sensory false perceptions. The person may or may not recognize those experiences as false. The hallucinations can be **auditory, visual, olfactory, gustatory, tactile,** or **somatic.** Hallucinations are commonly seen in schizophrenic patients. For example, hearing voices when alone in a room.

Hallucinatory voices are a common complaint reported by schizophrenic patients, although schizophrenia may present in a wide variety of forms. Table 6–6 provides a differential diagnosis of schizophrenia.

Review the following examples of written notes:

Perceptions: Hallucinations and illusions (−).

Perceptions: Hallucinatory voices present. No illusion.

Perceptions: Illusions; states that man in the painting of his dining room seems to be looking at him angrily.
Hallucinations: Visual (−), auditory (−).

Perceptions: He states experiencing auditory hallucination. Voices that come from other worlds and tell him to do things. No illusions were reported.

Thought

The **thought process** (T/P) is the way in which the person thinks. Assess how the patient organizes his thoughts in logical, relevant, and coherent form, as well as how he transmits them in terms of words and speech throughout the interview. Speech is like a window to a patient's mind. Describe the thought process as follows:

Flight of ideas (FOI)—a continuous flow of speech, accelerated, in which the patient jumps abruptly from one topic to another topic. FOI are seen during manic episodes, organized mental disorders, and schizophrenia.

Looseness of association (LOA)—ideas shift from one subject to another in an unrelated fashion. LOA is observed in schizophrenia, manic episodes, and other psychotic disorders.

TABLE 6–6. Schizophrenia: Differential Diagnosis and Criteria

Differential Diagnosis	Diagnostic Workup*
1. **Schizophrenia:** psychotic symptoms for at least 6 months, active phase for at least 1 week	1. CT scan of head
2. **Schizophreniform disorder:** like schizophrenia, but symptoms present for at least 1 month but less than 6 months	2. Urinary catecholamines (VMA)
3. **Brief psychotic disorder:** like schizophrenia, but symptoms present for at least 1 day but less than 1 month	3. Urinary toxicology studies
4. **Schizoaffective disorder:** like schizophrenia but with symptoms of mood disorder as well	4. CBC
5. **Paranoid personality disorder:** Similar to schizophrenia but without hallucinations and formal thought disorder	5. Electrolytes
6. **Delusional disorder:** Is characterized by non-bizarre delusions for at least one month, but lacks hallucinations, changes in affect, other thought disorders	
7. **Manic states**	
8. **Obsessive-compulsive disorder**	

CBC = complete blood count; CT = computed tomography; VMA = vanillylmandelic acid.
*It is not necessary to order every test; use your own criteria case by case.

Tangentiality—sudden changes in themes of conversation, such as replying to a question in an oblique or irrelevant way.

Circumstantiality—speech characterized by indirection and delay in reaching the point, and by inclusion of unnecessary detail, although the components of description are meaningfully connected. The speaker does not lose the point, as is characteristic of LOA, and clauses remain logically connected; however, to the listener, it seems that the end will never be reached. It is associated with schizophrenia mental and compulsive disorders.

Neologism—making up new words or condensed combination of several words coined by a person to express a highly complex idea not really understood by others.

Echolalia—repeating a word over and over.

Word salad—also known as incoherence; speech that is incoherent in terms of word order and grammar.

Blocking—a sudden interruption of speech in mid-sentence or before completion of an idea. This is seen in schizophrenia.

Clanging—speech characterized by the use of words in relation to sound and rhythm rather than meaning. Seen in schizophrenic and manic syndromes.

Thought content (T/C) is what the person is actually thinking about. Ask the patient/SP if there is any **particular idea** or problem that is affecting him or her at the time of the exam. Sometimes these are obvious and the patient/SP shows you that, openly. Sometimes you need to ask directly, looking for:

1. **Compulsions, obsessions, phobias, anxieties**
2. **Feelings of depersonalization,** which is the sense that one's self is different, changed, unreal, or that one has lost his or her identity
3. **Feelings unreality,** which is the sense that things in the environment are strange, unreal, or remote

4. **Delusions,** which are false beliefs not shared by others. These include delusions of persecution (e.g., the feeling of being followed by the CIA), grandiosity, jealous ideas, and reference (which is when the person believes that external events, objects, or people have a particular and unusual personal significance, such as believing that other people or the media are talking about him.)

Do not forget to question the patient about **suicidal ideation, intention, and plans.** The majority of patients who eventually kill themselves have told the examiner in one way or another about their desire to die. Table 6–7 lists the statistics and risk factors for suicide. Table 6–8 summarizes some behavioral disorders that the examiner may encounter in general practice.

See the following examples:

Thought

Thought process: Logical and goal directed(+), LOA(−), FOI(−), tangential(−) circumferential(−), concrete(−).

Thought content: Suicidal ideation(−), Homicidal ideation(−),

Delusions: Persecution (−), grandeur (−) and control (−).

Thought: Thought process showed some flight of ideas and occasional blocking. No delusions expressed.

Thought:

T/P: Coherent, logical, no FOI/LOA.

T/P: No suicidal or homicidal ideation.

Cognitive and Intellectual Functions

Evaluation of the cognitive functions is common. There are several tests, observations, and questions that give the examiner an idea of the cognitive and intellectual abilities of the patient/SP. The Mini-Mental Status Examination, better known as MMSE, produces a numerical score for this examination. The MMSE can be used in any other situation (e.g., in the neurologic exam or with geriatric patients) in which you consider it necessary to evaluate intellectual and cognitive function. The general evaluation addresses the following topics:

Level of consciousness. There are several types and levels of alertness:

Alert—the normal awake state

TABLE 6–7. Suicide and Risk Factors

Statistics on Suicide

8th leading cause of death in U.S. (Homicide ranks 12th; that is, more Americans kill themselves then are killed by others.)

3rd leading cause of death in people 15–24 years old (after accidents and homicide)

Rate of attempts in the U.S. is 11.3 per 100,000 persons (National Vital Statistics Report, 1998.)

Suicide attempts outnumber successful suicides

Risk Factors

Gender: Successful suicide is more common in men. Attempted suicide is more common in women. There is a 3:1 female-to-male ratio in suicide attempts.

Ethnicity: Whites have the highest rate of any race and ethnic group.

Religion: Highest among Protestants, followed by Jews and then Catholics.

Social: More common among single, unmarried, divorced, widowed, unemployed or retired

Occupation: Increased rate in professional women, particularly physicians. Among physicians, the rate is higher than for psychiatrists. Among other professionals, highest in dentists.

Associated factors: Mental health disorders such as mood and affective disorders. Alcohol is a factor in about 30% of all completed suicides. Eighteen percent of alcoholics die by suicide; according to the National Center of Health Statistics, 87% of these deaths are males.

TABLE 6-8. Other Behavioral Disorders

Anxiety Disorders	Somatoform Disorders	Eating Disorders	Factitious Disorders
1. Panic disorder	1. Somatization disorder	1. Anorexia nervosa	1. Factitious disorder
2. Phobias	2. Conversion disorder	2. Bulimia nervosa	2. Munchausen by proxy
3. Obsessive-compulsive disorder	3. Hypochondriasis		3. Malingering
4. Posttraumatic stress disorder	4. Pain disorder		
5. Generalized anxiety disorder	5. Body dysmorphic disorder		
Differential Diagnosis			
All of the above, *plus:*	All of the above, *plus:*	All of the above, *plus:*	All of the above, *plus:*
1. Somatization disorder	1. Anxiety disorder	1. Obesity	1. Somatization disorder
2. Anorexia nervosa	2. Major depression	2. Anxiety disorder	2. Conversion disorder
3. Schizophrenia	3. Psychotic disorder		3. Hypochondriasis
4. Drug and EtOH abuse			4. Pain disorder
Diagnostic Workup*			5. Any physical illness
1. IV sodium lactate	Order any general laboratory test that you consider relevant to the particular case presented to you during the CSA exam	1. CBC	
2. ECG/echocardiogram†		2. Electrolytes	These patients do not need any laboratory tests. Some of them may have highly sophisticated medical knowledge. They may ask you for invasive diagnostic tests, such as laparotomy.
		3. ESR	
		4. Urinalysis	
		5. BUN/Cr	
		6. TSH, T_4	
		7. Cholesterol	
		8. ECG, triceps skin-fold thickness	

BUN/Cr = blood urea nitrogen/creatine ratio; CBC = complete blood count; ECG = electrocardiogram; ESR = erythrocyte sedimentation rate; IV = intravenous; TSH = thyroid-stimulating hormone; T_4 = thyroxine.
*It is not necessary to order every diagnostic test; use your own criteria case by case.
†If you suspect mitral valve prolapse. (Mitral prolapse is associated with panic disorder in up to 50%.)

Distractible—easily distracted
Clouding—loss of ability to respond normally to external events.
Somnolence—abnormal sleepiness
Delirium—confusion, restlessness, disorientation, with anxiety and hallucinations
Stupor—little or no response to environmental stimuli
Coma—Total unconsciousness

Orientation is evaluated by skillful questioning in respect to **time, place,** and **person.** Questions about time, important dates, the patient's address, hospital location, own name, and names of relatives are sufficient. Disorientation occurs when memory and orientation are impaired, as in organic brain syndromes.

   Memory. Questions to the patient will determine remote and recent memory:

   Remote memory—Ask questions about birthdays, childhood, names of schools attended, past presidents, etc. Remote memory can be impaired in late stages of dementia.

   Recent memory—Ask about the events of the day, such as today's weather, lab tests taken, etc. Ask the SP to memorize three unrelated objects—for example, a name, an address, and the name of a plant. After 10 minutes ask him to repeat those things. Recent memory can be impaired in organic brain syndromes such as dementia, delirium and amnestic syndrome.

Concentration and attention. To measure this, use a digital repetition test. Ask the patient to subtract 7s serially from 100. Successful performance of this test depends on several factors, such as concentration, educational level, and IQ.

Capacity to read, write, and speak. Ask the patient to read a sentence and do what it says. Ask the patient/SP to write a sentence.

Visuospatial ability. Ask the patient to copy a figure, such as a circle, cross, rhombus, or cube. In the presence of intact vision and motor ability, poor performance in copying a figure suggest organic brain disease, such as dementia or parietal lobe damage.

Abstract thinking. Use similarities and proverb interpretation. Some examples include:

An orange and apple/Cat and mouse/ Paper and coal/ Piano and violin/ A church and a theater, etc.

A stitch in time saves nine/ A rolling stone gathers no moss/The proof of the pudding is in the eating/Don't count your chickens before they're hatched.

Concrete responses are given by patient/SPs with mental retardation, delirium, or dementia. Schizophrenics may respond concretely or with personal bizarre interpretations.

Fund of information and knowledge. Evaluate a patient's calculating ability, name of the past presidents, meaning of different words (e.g., apple, church, plural, etc.) and specific questions: *Where does the sun set? When is Labor Day? What are the names of the four seasons? How many days are in a week? How many things are in a dozen?*

It is not necessary to examine all parameters of this part of the MSE exam. Evaluate as the clinical condition of the patient/SP dictates. Again, your own criteria are important. The MMSE is a helpful alternative to this complex exam. Using this instrument, a skilled examination can be performed in 5 minutes.

One very common situation that may arise requires the examiner to differentiate between delirium and dementia. Table 6–9 reviews some important aspects about delirium and dementia.

Impulse Control

Impulse control is evaluated from the history or the patient's behavior during the interview. Describe how the patient reacts to the environment and how he or she controls emotions. Patients with impulse control disorders are unable to resist an impulse. Before the act they have increased anxiety, and while committing the act they feel pleasure. Studies have reported some alterations in the serotonergic system mediators that appear to be related to the following impulse disorders:

Intermittent explosive disorder. This disorder is characterized by episodes of failure to resist aggressive impulses that result in serious assaultive acts or destruction of property. Usually a stressor exists, and can be resolved quickly. Consider trauma, seizures, hyperactivity. Treat with selective serotonin reuptake inhibitor (SSRI) drugs.

Kleptomania. This disorder is associated with brain diseases and mild mental retardation. Treat with psychotherapy and SSRI drugs.

Pyromania. This disorder is linked with cruelty to animals and antisocial traits. Manage with behavioral treatment.

Pathological gambling. This is associated with alcoholism, exposure to gambling, attention deficit hyperactivity disorder, obsessive-compulsive and panic disorders. Treat with psychotherapy.

Trichotillomania. This disorder links with obsessive-compulsive, depressive, and borderline disorders. It is common in adolescents. Manage with behavioral treatment and SSRI drugs.

See the following examples:

Impulse control: Normal

Impulse control: Aggressive

TABLE 6–9. Delirium and Dementia

	Delirium	Dementia
Etiology		
Cerebral causes	Brain trauma, encephalitis, epilepsy, meningitis, subarachnoid bleeding	Alzheimer disease, brain trauma, cerebral hypoxia, Huntington disease
Somatic causes	Arrhythmias, electrolyte imbalances, hepatic encephalopathy, hypoxia, hypotension, uremia, thiamine deficiency	Intracranial tumors, Korsakoff syndrome, multi-infarct dementia, Pick disease, multiple sclerosis
External causes	Alcohol, anticonvulsants, insulin, hypnotics, opiates, PCP, steroids, CO narcosis, anticholinergics, etc.	
Onset		
	Acute	Insidious
Characteristics		
	Recent memory very impaired	Recent memory more impaired than remote memory
	Usually reversible state	Usually *not* reversible state
	Visual hallucinations very common	Hallucinations not common. Sundowning is common. This is a cognitive diurnal variable effect: patients are worse at night and early morning.
	Arousal, stupor, or agitation	Normal level of arousal
	Consciousness impaired	Consciousness not impaired
	Orientation impaired	
	Orientation impaired initially	Orientation intact initially
Differential Diagnosis		
	All of the above, *plus:*	All of the above, *plus:*
	Delirium	Delirium
	Dementia	Dementia
	Pseudodementia	Pseudodementia
		Thyroid diseases
Diagnostic Workup		
	1. CT scan of head	1. Physical exam and neurological exam + MSE
	2. CBC	2. B_{12} and folate levels
	3. Electrolytes	3. Rapid plasma reaginin
	4. ABG	4. CBC
	5. ECG	5. Electrolytes
	6. Blood drug screen	6. ABG
		7. TSH, T3, T4
		8. CT/MRI of the head

ABG = arterial blood gases; CBC = complete blood count; CT = computed tomography; ECG = electrocardiogram; MRI = magnetic resonance imaging; MSE = mental status examination; T_3 = triiodothyronine; T_4 = thyroxine; TSH = thyroid-stimulating hormone.

Judgment and Insight

Judgment is the use of common sense to resolve problems of daily life (e.g., *What can you do when you run out of medicine?*)

Insight is the ability of the patient to act appropriately and react to the nature and extent of the current difficulties and their ramifications in his or her daily life. Be explicit, as shown in the following examples:

Judgment and Insight: *Good*
Judgment: *Poor*
Insight: *Fair*
Judgment: *Good*
Insight: *Fair*

Finally, review the following examples of the overall MSE, writing medical notes as you will on the day of the CSA exam. Keep in mind that in the following medical notes (+) present and (−) means absent. Psychiatrists write their medical notes as you see in these examples. Although you can write out "present" or "absent," during the CSA you may want to save time.

Mental Status Examination (patient with bipolar I disorder, recently depressed)

Appearance: Satisfactorily groomed, appearing stated age
Attitude: Cooperative
Activity (motor): Appropriate, good eye contact
Articulation (speech): Fluent, normal rate, tone, and volume
Mood: Euthymic
Affect: Appropriate
Thought process: Logical and goal-directed, looseness of association (LOA) (−), flight of ideas (FOI) (−), tangential (−), circumferential (−), concrete(−).
Thought content:
Suicidal ideation (−)
Homicidal ideation (−)
Hallucination: auditory (−), visual (−), tactile (−)
Delusions: persecution (−), grandeur (−), control (−)
Sensorium: Sleepy and oriented to person, place and time
Concentration and memory: Normal
Insight and judgment: Good

MSE (Patient with alcohol dependence)

Lying in bed, somewhat suspicious. Poor grooming. Attentive, guarded. Fair eye contact. Speech normal rate, rhythm, tone, volume. No psychomotor agitation/retardation/abnormal movements. Mood irritable, affect congruent, somewhat labile. T/P, coherent, logical, no FOI/LOA. Insight fair, judgment poor. Memory intact. Intellect average.

Mental Status Exam (Patient with intermittent explosive disorder who recently hit his wife)

Pt appears somewhat suspicious. He looks well groomed and is cooperative. Eye contact is good. Speech normal in fluency, tonality, and quality.
Mood: Depressed
Affect: Appropriate
T/P: Apparently normal
T/C: Suicidal ideation (+), homicidal ideation (−), compulsions (−)
Patient states that he cannot have self-control over himself after minor discussions with his wife. Delusions (−). Insight and judgment are good. Impulse control normal during the interview.

MINI MENTAL STATUS EXAMINATION (MMSE)

The Mini Mental Status Examination (MMSE) is an abbreviated instrument that helps you evaluate the patient's cognitive and intellectual functions. The MMSE produces a numerical score, with up to 30 points given for every correct answer to questions, that provides a guide to the patient's probable diagnosis (e.g., likely organic, < 27). The MMSE can be given systematically to any patient as a screening tool of the cognitive and intellectual functions. One important aspect is that with the MMSE you can have an objective parameter. The MMSE is used not only for psychiatric evaluation—it also can be used for other clinical conditions, such as nervous system examination or assessment of the competence of elderly patients. Review the following medical notes and see Table 6–10 for a description of the MMSE.

The following two examples use different forms of MSE, including the MMSE. As stated before, note that the MMSE can be used not only for psychiatric patients but also for other clinical conditions that mandate this kind of evaluation. Finally, note the use of the multiaxial system under the psychiatric notes. (This system might not be helpful on the CSA exam, however.)

MMSE Under Psychiatric-oriented Case

> Lying in bed in lateral supine position. Normal grooming, attentive, guarded. Good eye contact. Speech normal in rate, rhythm, tone, and volume. No psychomotor agitation, retardation, or abnormal movements. Mood irritable, affect congruent, somewhat labile. MMSE 30/30.

TABLE 6–10. Mini-Mental Status Examination (MMSE)

Category	Points
1. **Level of consciousness:** Awake, clouding of consciousness or unconsciousness	0–3
2. **Orientation:** To time, place, and person. One point for every correct parameter.	0–3
3. **Attention and calculation:** Serial 7s. One point for every correct subtraction.	0–3
4. **Registration:** Patient names 3 objects, then is asked to repeat them. One point for every correct answer (ec/a)	0–3
5. **Visuospatial ability:** Patient is asked to copy a figure.	0–3
6. **Memory/recall:** Recent, remote, recent past, and immediate retention. Ask for the names of the three objects asked in question 4. One point for each correct answer (ec/a).	0–3
7. **Language, naming and repetition:** Point to an object, then ask patient to name it. Have the patient repeat "No, ifs, ands, or buts." Obey orders such as "close your eyes." One point ec/a	0–3
8. **Three-stage command:** Instruct patient to take a piece of paper in his or her right hand, fold the paper in half, and put the paper on the floor. Give 3 points if patient follows instructions correctly.	0–3
9. **Abstract thinking:** Similarities and proverb interpretation.	0–3
10. **Capacity to read and write:** Ask the patient to read something, write a sentence, and do what it says or explain the meaning of the entire sentence.	0–3
	Maximum Points: 30

(Adapted with permission from Perkin E, Cookson DB: *Pocket Guide to Clinical Examination,* 2nd ed. Times Mirror, 1997, p 195.)

MMSE Under Neurological-oriented Case

> Speech, normal fluency and coherent. The patient is alert and oriented × 3. Mini Mental Exam 24/30, minus for memory and abstract thinking. Cranial nerves (CN) II-XII are grossly within normal limits. Motor, sensory, and reflexes are normal.

The following example illustrates notes from a multiaxial system assessment. (For CSA purposes, the multiaxial system will not be helpful; therefore, depending on the time you have, you may want to skip this section.)

Impressions

> Axis I: Schizophrenic disorder, paranoid type
> Axis II: No diagnosis
> Axis III: CAD, IDDM, HTN. Post-MI.
> Axis IV: Relapsed on symptoms, separated from his wife
> Axis V: GAF 35

A/P

> Axis I: Alcohol dependence
> Axis II: Deferred
> Axis III: Esophageal varices, HBcAb +, alcoholic liver cirrhosis
> Axis IV: Unknown
> Axis V: GAF 40

A/Plan

> Axis I: Partner relational problem
> Axis II: No dx
> Axis III: None
> Axis IV: Unemployment
> Axis V: GAF 83, highest level the past year

DIFFERENTIAL DIAGNOSIS

Notes for the differential diagnosis are done in the same way as in the general exam.

DIAGNOSTIC WORKUP

Notes for the diagnostic workup are done the same way as those for the general exam.

7

Pediatrics: Writing Medical Notes

INTRODUCTION

The specialty of pediatrics covers the years from birth through adolescence. When you assess an infant or a child, you must remember that the patient is still growing and developing. The ECFMG® has recently become more specific about pediatric cases on the CSA exam and the current policy is that **there are no children presenting as standardized patients (SPs).** However, there may be cases dealing with pediatric issues in which you encounter the parent or caregiver of a sick child. In these cases, physical examination of the child is obviously not possible and will not be expected (Candidate Orientation Manual, ECFMG®, 2001). However, we can be sure that you will encounter an *adolescent patient* on the CSA exam. *How old will the youngest adolescent SP be that you may encounter?* This is a very difficult question to answer, but we can assume that all SPs are adults, and some SPs are young adults simulating being a high-school age adolescent or so.

The key to success is the same as before: Pretend you are in a real clinical situation. We can be sure that you will encounter an adolescent patient on the CSA exam. Being prepared to confront any situation is the best tool for success.

This chapter provides a complete review of the information on pediatrics you will need for the CSA exam.

GENERAL

The goal of health supervision for every child is to achieve optimal growth and development. Tracking the history of growth and development is very important. The pediatric history usually is obtained from a second person—usually a parent—and consequently is subject to the memory or precision of the person who informs you of the reason for the office visit. However, never forget the value of the child as an informant. It may take time to win the confidence of young children. Inspection and observation are important tools. In general, pediatric notes follow the same format as those for adult patients, but the manner and order in which they are approached differ, and the emphasis is different in children. In this chapter, it is impossible to cover a complete pediatric medical history as would be needed in real clinical practice. In addition, some cases that are presented to you in this book are unlikely to be presented to you during the CSA exam. This chapter focuses only on the notes that may be relevant for the CSA exam.

GROWTH AND DEVELOPMENT

Growth is an increase in size or in the number of cells of the tissue, organs, or systems. **Development** means an increment in the specialization of function of the different organs and systems. The continuum of growth from birth to adulthood has been described by three main phases: infancy, childhood, and adolescence. Table 7–1 describes infancy and childhood. It is important to note the developmental milestones that help us to determine the presence of any psychomotor or intellectual retardation.

Normal patterns of development encompass a wide range of variations. For convenience, development usually is considered under eight general categories: gross motor, fine motor, behavioral, vision, hearing, expression in language, comprehension of language, and social skills. Not every category is necessarily pertinent in every case.

Infancy

Infancy is the time **from birth to 2 years of age.** Two key factors that can affect development during this stage are **nutrition** and **hormones,** which control the infant's metabolism. Infancy can be divided into three stages: **newborn** (birth to 2 weeks); **early infancy** (2 weeks to 6 months); and **late infancy** (6 months to 2 years). At birth, infants have inherent reflexes such as the Moro reflex, the palmar reflex, the Babinski reflex, and the rooting reflex. These reflexes disappear by the ages of 2 months (palmar grasp), 3–6 months (Moro reflex), and 12 months (Babinski reflex). The most important task for the physician in early infancy is educating the parents on feeding, sleep habits, safety, and disease prevention and immunizations. During late infancy, dental care, immunizations, self-feeding, toilet training, and sleep habits are emphasized.

Childhood

Childhood is defined as the period **from 2 years to 11 years of age.** This phase can be divided into **preschool years** (2–5 years of age) and **school years** (5–11 years). During the preschool years the same emphasis as for infancy applies. Play, control of television viewing, control of computer "chatting" and playing, transfer of attachment from home to school, and school learning will be very important points of discussion with parents. During the school years, sex education and attention to the child's own health habits will be important.

Adolescence

Adolescence runs from **puberty until the achievement of final adult stature** (12–20 years old). Key points of discussion with the adolescent are as follows:

Sexual activity: *Are you sexually active right now? Are you using birth control? Are you aware of the risks of sexually transmitted disease? What are your plans for starting your own family someday?*

Substance abuse: *Do you ever get high?*

Mental health: *Do you ever get down or depressed?*

Home situation and self image: *How do you feel when you look in the mirror every morning?*

It is very important to reassure the adolescent patient that any information that he or she provides to you will be confidential.

PEDIATRIC MEDICAL HISTORY

The key point to remember is that there are important differences between ages, but the pediatric note format is almost the same for all age groups. (We try not to repeat

TABLE 7–1. Growth and Development from Birth to Age 12

Phase	Motor Skills	Developmental Issues	Language Skills	Common Problems	Procedures (Other)
Newborn (birth 28 days)					
	Reflexes Palmar grasp Moro reflex Babinski reflex	Starts socialization, can follow (track) human face Reflexive smile (at birth) Attachment Unpredictable demands	Crying	Rashes Conjunctivitis Weight loss Jaundice Breastfeeding problems	Prophylaxis of gonococcal ophthalmia. Vitamin K (0.5–1.0 mg) Metabolic screening **Phenylke-tonuria** **Hypothy roidism** Galactosemia Cystic fibrosis Hg electrophore-sis or solubility test
Early infancy (28 days–6 months)					
	Sits with support at 4 mos Rolls over Grasps a rattle Places objects in the mouth By 6 mos, transfers a toy from one hand to another. By 2 mos can lift the head 45°	From unpredict-able to predict-able demands Social smile (5–8 wks) Attachment Parent–child synchrony Localizes sounds Tracks human face	Babbles and coos	Dacryostenosis Diaper rashes Generic Candidal Ulcerative Impetigo Seborrheic Colic Constipation Teething begins at about 6 mos.	Immunizations (completed at 6 months) **DTP—3 doses** **TOPV—3 doses** **Hib—3 doses** Metabolic screen-ing: repeat PKU and hypothy-roidism For infants fed breast milk only: **Vitamin D 400IU/day** **Fluoride 0.25 mg/day** For infants fed only formula· **No supple-ments re-quired** Begin vision and hearing screen-ing
Late infancy (6 m–2 years)					
	Sits alone well at 9–10 months Can hold own weight with legs Crawls, creeps when prone Walking at 1 year At 18 mos, descends, and by 2 y walks up stairs unaided	Starts to explore the environ-ment Uses pincer finger **(6–12m);** pincer grasp at 15 months By 9–10 m feeds self finger food Can stack four blocks and hold a cup securely by 2 years.	Dada, Mama **(9–10 m)** Uses 1–5 words **(12–15 months)** Uses pronouns, combines two words in short sentences **(2 y):** What's this? Decreased appetite	Tantrums Night crying Stranger and separation anxiety **(1.5 y)** Decreased appetite Teething*	Immunizations: **MMR, DTP, TOPV** and **Hib** vaccines Screening: **Anemia (at 1 y)** **Lead poisoning** **Tuberculosis** (PPD only for patients at risk) Dental care and fluoride.

continued

TABLE 7–1. Growth and Development from Birth to Age 12 *Continued*

Phase	Motor Skills	Developmental Issues	Language Skills	Common Problems	Procedures (Other)
Preschool (2–5 years)					
	Rough-and-tumble play Pedals a tricycle at 3 years	Parallel play at 2 years Group play at 3 years Birth of sibling may cause **sibling rivalry** Attachment starts to decrease as school approaches. Separation is important. Gender identity fixed at around 4–5 years. By 3 y can draw a vertical line, copy a circle. By 3–4 y can copy a cross, square, diamond, etc.	Uses routine sentences by age 3 years Can point to parts of the body as waist, knee, etc. Responds to questions such as name, age, address, etc.	Separation anxiety Sibling rivalry Night awakenings Stuttering	Immunizations: booster doses of **DTP, TOPV** at **4–5y** Screening: **Vision** at 3–4 years **Hearing** at 4 years **Urinalysis** once bladder control attained **Anemia Cholesterol** at 2 y, if + family history Measure blood pressure (recommended at 3 y)
School-age (5–12 years)					
	Increasingly complex tasks such as skipping, hopping on one foot, etc. 6-year-old child can tie shoelaces.	Able to write and draw (5 y). Prefers to play with children of the same sex **(latency)** Autonomy: by age of 8 y, **peers** become more important than family. Child acquires logical thought. By the age of 8 he is able to establish hierarchies, logical relationships, etc. **Formal operations** developed[†]	Able to read, write and spell words.	Confrontations with teachers, parents due to peer influence Separation anxiety Recurrent pains Poor school performance	Immunizations: Booster dose of **MMR** at 11–12 y Screenings: **Vision Hearing Urinalysis Cholesterol** (if positive FH)

DTP = diphtheria + tetanus toxoids + pertussis; Hib = *Haemophilus influenzae* type b; MMR= measles, mumps, and rubella; TOPV = total oral poliovirus.
*Begins at 6 m, excessive drooling and rhinorrhea.
[†]At 12 y starts to use hypothetical and abstract thinking.

information already explained, so only important aspects specific to pediatrics will be mentioned during the course of this chapter.) Figure 7–1 shows the general structure of the pediatric exam.

PEDIATRIC HISTORY

Chief Complaint (CC)

The chief complaint section follows the same format as that for adult notes (see Chapter 3). Use the patient, parent, or guardian's own words about the case.

See the following examples:

Chief Complaint

Joe is a 12 yo boy with IDDM who is admitted because of altered mental status.

Chief Complaint

Bryce is a 2 yo boy admitted due to irritability. Patient's mother stated on presentation that the patient had become more irritable since the motor vehicle accident.

C.C.

This is a 3 yo boy who came showing irritability and abdominal discomfort. Mother states that he had a fever of 100°F, diarrhea and abdominal pain.

CC

Patient's mother stated on presentation that the patient had become noticeably more irritable since the accident.

A) PEDIATRIC MEDICAL HISTORY
1. Chief complaint (CC)
2. History of the present illness (HPI)
3. Past medical history (PMH)
   ···► *Birth history*
       + Prenatal, natal, and neonatal history
   ···► *Feeding history*
   ···► *Growth and development*
   ···► *Immunizations and*
       screening procedures
   ···► *Childhood illnesses*
   ···► *Social development*
4. Social history (SH)
5. Family history (FH)
6. Review of systems (ROS)

B) PHYSICAL EXAMINATION
1. General examination (GE)
2. HEENT
3. Neck
4. Chest ···► *Respiratory system*
      ···► *Heart*
5. Abdomen
6. Genital/inguinal examination
7. Neurologic
8. Musculoskeletal

C) DIFFERENTIAL DIAGNOSIS
–Plans for dif. diagnosis (1-5)

D) DIAGNOSTIC WORKUP
–Plans for diagnosis (1-5)
–Plans for rectal/pelvic/female breast

FIGURE 7–1. Format for a pediatric note.

History of the Present Illness (HPI)

History of the present illness follows the adult format. It is the history of the **present illness,** not the history of all illnesses. Information to be elicited includes when the problem started, how members of the family responded to the patient's symptoms and concerns, and whether the problem has any relation to particular events. See the following examples:

History of the Present Illness

The patient's mother stated that the patient was well until yesterday evening, when she noticed excessive crying, ↓ appetite, ↑ T°, vomiting ×2, and diarrhea ×4. She states that they recently traveled to Mexico by car to visit family there. No other relatives in home were sick.

Hx of the Present Illness

The patient's mother stated that Mike was well until this morning, when he reported dysuria, urgency and ↑ in frequency, and fever. Vesicoureteral reflux was diagnosed one year ago.

HPI

The pt reported having been treated with topical clindamycin and Benzoyl peroxide due to acne 3 weeks ago. He was relatively well until the past week when he noted the appearance of pustules and inflamed comedones. He is very upset because his peers in school constantly make jokes about him.

HPI

Joyce refers having pain in her R. ear, especially at night and when someone touches it. She was well until yesterday evening when she started having cold-like symptoms.

PAST MEDICAL HISTORY (PMH)

The past medical history is a broad section that differs significantly from the adult medical notes. You need to include a chronological description of the child's physical development—normal or abnormal—from conception until the present time. Include any preventive measures or screening tests performed on the child. There is no single format that you need to follow on every pediatric patient. You need to formulate your questions according to the CC, the child's age, and available time. As with any other situations, being precise and concise in your notes and questions is always helpful. The general format includes the following information:

> **Birth History:** This part is particularly important during the first 2 years of life, especially because of possible repercussions on possible future neurologic and developmental problems. Divide your descriptions as follows:
>
> **Prenatal:** Include information about maternal health before and during the pregnancy. *Did the mother receive adequate prenatal care?* List details about nutrition, specific illnesses or complications during the pregnancy (weight gain, vaginal bleeding), *medications, smoking?, alcohol?,* duration of pregnancy, attitudes toward the pregnancy and the coming child and responsibility.
>
> **Natal:** Place of birth, nature of labor and delivery, including degree of difficulty and complications encountered. Birth order and birth weight.
>
> **Neonatal:** *Did the baby cry immediately after birth? What were the Apgar scores?*

Were any resuscitation efforts necessary? Note gestational age, any congenital abnormalities, and any specific problems with cyanosis, respiratory distress, jaundice, convulsions, anemia, infections, and feeding.

Feeding history: This category is very important during the first 2 years of life. Always remember that breast milk is the optimal source of infant nutrition and commercially prepared formula is only an acceptable alternative. For study purposes we classify the feeding history as follows:

Infancy: Describe the type of feeding the baby received. For breast-fed babies, ask about the frequency, duration, and the use (or not) of supplementary artificial formulas or vitamins from breast or bottle to cup. For formula-fed babies, ask about the type, concentration, amount, frequency, difficulties, and method of weaning. Describe the use of supplements such as vitamins or iron. Finally, describe the time and introduction of **solid foods** and any problem encountered with them.

Childhood: Describe the child's general dietary habits, what the child likes or dislikes, and usage of salt. A general description of the type of diet on a weekly period will be useful to give you a better idea of the child's nutritional status.

Growth and development: This part of the clinical history helps to determine whether physical growth and developmental milestones are being met, and to determine whether there is any growth delay or psychomotor or intellectual retardation. Check the weight, height, and head circumference as follows: always obtain height and weight at every child visit and compare it every 2 years; head circumference at 2–4 weeks and 2, 4, 6, 8, and 12 months. Always, when possible, compare previous medical records and all measurements with standard growth charts. (Although some of these recommendations are not helpful for the actual CSA exam, always keep them in mind in case you need to provide advice to the parent SP.) Developmental milestones should be written down, such as the age at which the child held up his or her head while prone, when he or she first rolled over, sat without support, and so forth (see Table 7–1).

Immunizations: Note the date of administration of each vaccine, scheduled boosters, etc. Table 7–2 shows the recommended immunization schedule for healthy infants and children.

Screening procedures: Write the dates and results of the most relevant information about screening tests such as vision, hearing, PPD, hematocrit, etc. (Table 7–1 lists recommended ages for screening tests.)

Childhood illnesses: Write down what illnesses the child has had: measles, chickenpox, mumps, etc. See Table 7–3 for the differential diagnosis of childhood illnesses.

Medications: Self-explanatory.

TABLE 7–2. Recommended Immunization Schedules

Age	Vaccine
2 months	DTP, TOPV, Hib, hepatitis
4 months	DTP, TOPV, Hib, hepatitis
6 months	DTP, TOPV, Hib, hepatitis
15 months	MMR, Hib
18 months	DTP, TOPV
4–6 years	DTP, TOPV
11–12 years	DTP, TOPV, MMR
14–16 years	Td

DTP = diphtheria, tetanus toxoids, and pertussis;; Hib = *Haemophilus influenzae* type b; MMR= measles, mumps, and rubella; Td = tetanus toxoid (adult); TOPV = total oral poliovirus.

TABLE 7–3. Differential Diagnosis of Childhood Illnesses

Rubella	Measles	Roseola Infantum	Erythema Infectiosum	Varicella and Zoster	Scarlet Fever
Other Names					
German measles	Rubeola	Exanthem subitum	Fifth disease	Chickenpox, shingles*	
Etiology					
Rubella virus	Paramyxovirus	Herpesvirus 6	Human parvovirus	Herpes zoster virus†	Erythrogenic toxin‡
Clinical Features					
Risk of congenital infection§ No clinical symptoms Posterior auricular cervical lymph node Maculopapular rash on face, and generalized	Erythematous maculopapular rash begins on the head and spreads downward, in 4–5 resolves from the head downward Conjunctivitis Koplik spots Complications include laryngitis, croup, pneumonia, encephalitis, gastroenteritis, and hepatitis	Abrupt fever of 39–41°C After 4 days, papulomacular rash appears on the trunk and spreads peripherally Leukocytosis as high as 20 K Then leukopenia, neutropenia Major cause of febrile seizures	No prodrome Low or absent fever Rash—erythema on cheeks ("slapped face" sign) Erythematous maculopapular rash that invades arms and then goes to the trunk and legs	Varicella is highly contagious, occurring in children. Self-limited Characterized by pruritic rash, first on the trunk, peripherally begins as papules and then into tear-drop vesicles Low-grade fever	Pharyngitis is accompanied by erythematous rash that is finely punctate of minute papules, giving a characteristic "sand paper" texture to the skin Rash is initially on the upper trunk, generalized, but sparing the palms and soles Face looks flushed, "strawberry tongue" (enlarged papilla on a coated tongue) Accentuation of the rash in the skin folds (Pastia lines)
Diagnosis					
CBC may show leukopenia and atypical lymphocytes ELISA for IgG and IgM antibodies‖	CBC may show lymphopenia, neutropenia Immuno-fluorescent staining of a smear of respiratory secretions for measles antigen Enzyme immuno-assay	Clinical picture and CBC	Clinical picture and CBC	Clinical picture Tzanck test# FAMA test ELISA test PCR	Clinical picture *Streptococcus* species isolated on throat Anti-streptolysin O CBC
Therapy					
Self-limited	Supportive	Self-limited	Supportive	Supportive	Penicillin

continued

TABLE 7–3. Differential Diagnosis of Childhood Illnesses *Continued*

Rubella	Measles	Roseola Infantum	Erythema Infectiosum	Varicella and Zoster	Scarlet Fever
Prevention					
Live attenuated vaccine	Alone or as MMR vaccine.			Varicella vaccine	

CBC = complete blood count; ELISA = enzyme-linked immunosorbent assay; FAMA = fluorescent antibody to membrane antigen; IgG = immunoglobulin G; IgM = immunoglobulin M; MMR = measles, mumps, and rubella; PCR = polymerase chain reaction.
*Shingles are caused by herpes zoster virus.
†**HZV** that affects sensory nerves and is more common in adults.
‡**Erythrogenic toxin,** which are currently designated as streptococcal pyrogenic enterotoxins A, B, and C.
§Characterized by deafness, cataracts, glaucoma, congenital heart disease, mental retardation.
∥Acute rubella is diagnosed by observing 4-fold or greater increase in the titer of IgG antibodies between acute phase and convalescent phase, or by observing the presence of IgM antibody in a single acute phase serum sample. In pregnant women, the presence of IgM antibody indicates recent infection, whereas a 1:8 or greater titer of IgG antibody indicates immunity and then protection of the fetus.
#Performed by taking scrapings from the base of the vesicle that demonstrate multinucleated giant cells with intranuclear inclusions that indicate varicella, herpes zoster, or herpes simplex infection.

Allergies: Pay attention to problems common in infancy, such as urticaria, eczema, allergic rhinitis, reactions to medications, hypersensitivities, etc.

Operations, injuries, hospitalizations: Note any particular event according to parent report, including any complications, when it occurred, length of hospitalization, etc.

Social development: This is broad information that you can approach in different parts of the interview and clinical examination, but you also need to question the parents in a general manner and mention anything in your notes that you consider it necessary. Ask about the following topics, focusing only on important information related to the chief complaint. You can complement this part with information from Table 7–1.

Sleep: Ask what time the child goes to bed, his or her sleep pattern, whether child has nightmares, terrors, etc.

Toileting: Age when the child gains bowel and bladder control. Methods used to train him/her. *Any problems? Enuresis or encopresis? Bedwetting?*

Speech: Review speech development (see Table 7–1). *Stuttoring?* Any other problems? etc.

Habits: Thumb sucking, pacifier use, pica, nailbiting, ritualistic behavior, headbanging, etc.

Discipline: Ask about child behavior, responsibilities, temperament, response to adult orders, temper tantrums, etc.

Schooling: Describe the childcare experience, nursery school, kindergarten (age of entrance), adjustment on entry, academic achievement.

Sexuality: Questions vary depending on age. In general, ask about conception and pregnancy (parent's response to child), girl and boy differences, masturbation, menstruation, nocturnal emissions, and so forth.

Personality: Relationship with parents, siblings, and peers. Level of independence, activities, personal interests, etc.

Review the following examples:

Past Medical History *(Infant patient)*

Mother reports that she had no prenatal, natal, or neonatal problems. Mother also states that baby cried instantly after the delivery. Weaning at 11 months, immunizations up to date, no allergies, she walks alone since 1 year old, 4 months ago; plays with other children.

PMH *(Adolescent patient)*

Tonsillectomy at 6 yo, appendectomy at 13 yo. He denies other special problems during infancy and childhood. He is up to date with immunizations. He started to smoke 1 year ago, half a pack/day, he reports smoking marijuana with high school peers sporadically. He doesn't have any future plans to continue college studies.

PMHx

Mother states that she consumed large amounts of EtOH during pregnancy. She also reports that her baby was hospitalized after birth for 3 weeks, baby also underwent cleft palate surgery at 2 years old. Pt had feeding problems due to his birth defect. Immunizations ok, varicella at 3 yo, no allergies. He plays with friends, no separation anxiety reported, he speaks several sentences with some nasal predomination phonation.

Social History (SH)

Get a brief description of the child's life environment. Describe how the house or apartment is set up, number of bedrooms, location (neighborhood, city, rural), etc. Find out if the child has his or her own bedroom, and ask if there is an air conditioner and heater. Describe the parents' occupations and level of education. Does the mother work outside the home?

See the following medical note examples:

Social History

Charles lives with both parents and his 12 yo sister. He has his own bedroom. The house is in a middle-class neighborhood. Both parents have a college education. At the present time only the father works outside the home, at City Memorial Hospital.

SH

Kiara lives with her mother and three siblings: 2 brothers and 1 sister, ages 16, 12, and 8. She lives in a poor neighborhood in the southeast section of the city. Her mother is a single mother, welfare-dependent, who works sporadically cleaning apartments.

SH

This adolescent pt comes from a disrupted family. His childhood has been spent split between his parents. He has half brothers from both parents. At this time he works part-time at a fast food restaurant. He states that he is saving money for his college studies.

Family History (FH)

The family history follows a similar format to that in adult notes. Take the most pertinent information about any problems of or between the child's parents. Note the parents' ages, consanguinity, general health information, height, weight, etc. Note the number of the mother's pregnancies, and number of actual siblings. Document potential hereditary problems such as obesity, NIDDM, HTN, cancer, etc. Use the format that suits you best (writing or diagrammatic format). For genetic inherited disorders, the diagrammatic format is more explanatory.

See the following examples of written notes:

Family History

Father and mother alive and healthy. They are 30 and 27 years old, respectively, grandfather 67 years old with well-controlled NIDDM, grandmother died of breast cancer at the age of 48. No other problems in first-degree relatives were reported. This is the first child in the family and no previous pregnancies were reported.

Family History

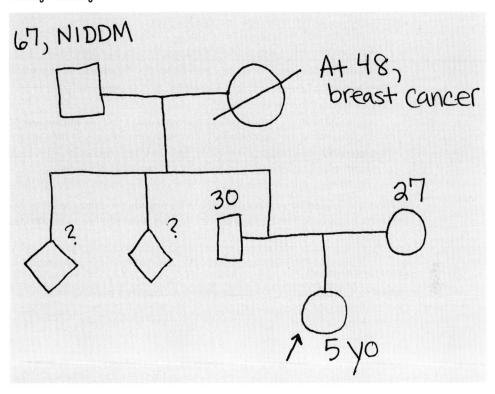

Review of Systems (ROS)

The amount of attention paid to the review of systems varies depending on how much time you have. You can merely make a checklist of the systems that you have already asked about during the visit. You can follow the same format described under ROS on an adult medical note. This part of the exam helps you catch some data that you might have missed during previous visits. Suit your questions to the child's age. See examples of general written medical notes for adults in Chapter 3.

PHYSICAL EXAMINATION

As explained, this chapter focuses on the most important aspects of the pediatric examination from early infancy through adolescence. The physical examination is a very important part of the medical history. Some aspects are similar to those for adult patients, but for some the emphasis varies depending on the child's age. Again, no children will be presenting as SPs during the CSA exam. An encounter (e.g., with the parent of a sick child) will not be able to include a physical examination of the child. However, be prepared to answer any question that the parent or caretaker may have about his or her child.

General Examination (GE)

The general survey permits you to obtain an overview of the patient's health without focusing on a particular organ or system. This section covers the measurements of vital signs and somatic growth, which is particularly important in infants and children. One important thing to remember is that blood pressure measurements often are omitted. For CSA purposes, you will not be able to take blood pressure from a child, because a child will not be present (see ECFMG® policy explained before). Be prepared to order or recommend it to the parent or caretaker. In general practice, **blood pressure screening is recommended on a yearly basis from ages 3 to 20.** Remember the normal variations with age (see Table 7-4).

Somatic growth measurement is a very important aspect during infancy and childhood to help determine any problem with delayed physical growth. It is recommended to check the child's weight, height, and head circumference at the following intervals:

Head circumference: At 2–4 weeks, 2, 4, 6, 8, 12 months.

Chest circumference: Sometimes used (especially in newborns) as a comparative measure for head size. Head size should exceed chest circumference until the age of 2 years and be smaller than the chest circumference thereafter.

Weight and height: At 2–4 weeks, 2,4, 6, 8, 12, and 18 months, and at 2, 3, 4, 5, 6 years (and then every 2 years until 20 years old). Whenever possible, these values should be compared with previous medical records (in a real clinical practice).

See the following examples. (Note: During these examples that the term toddler refers to a child who is 15 months to 2 1/2 years of age, and you would not see an SP who is a toddler during the CSA exam.)

General Examination

Mildly ill-appearing toddler with apparent respiratory distress.
T: 37°C, P: 140/min, R: 45 resp/min.

General Exam

An apparently normal full-term male newborn.
T: 38°C, P: 140/min, R: 30 resp/min.
Somatic Growth: H: 50 cm, W: 3070 g, HC: 36 cm, CC: 32 cm.

General Examination

Mildly ill-appearing, no apparent distress observed.
T: 39.5°C, BP: 130/85 mm Hg, P: 100/min, R: 28 resp/min
Somatic Growth: Height 95 cm, weight 30 kg.

HEENT

This part of the clinical examination includes the evaluation of the head, eyes, ears, nose, and throat, better known as HEENT. This part follows the same format as adult medical written notes, but some differences apply.

Head. As a quick review, the newborn's head accounts for 1/4 of body length and 1/3 of body weight. The anterior fontanelle is the largest at birth and normally closes between 4 and 26 months; the posterior fontanelle closes by 2 months of age. Remember that the sutures can be felt as smoothly depressed ridges and the fontanelles as soft concavities. If there is any increase in the tenseness and constant fullness seen and felt in the anterior fontanelle, suspect an increase in the intracranial pressure (ICP). The tenseness of the fontanelle may vary if the child cries, coughs, or vomits. When the child is dehydrated—for example, secondary to gastroenteritis—the fontanelle can be felt to be depressed on palpation. Pulsations sometimes can be felt through palpation. Note any asymmetry of the skull and face. Percuss the head by tapping your index finger over the head surface. The **cracked-pot sound,** which occurs when you percuss the parietal bone prior to closure of the sutures, and **Chvostek sign,** elicited when you percuss at the top of the cheek just below the zygomatic bone, producing a contraction of the facial muscle in the immediate area, are normal findings on normal newborns. (In adults, it may indicate hypocalcemia or tetany). Finally, transilluminate and auscultate the head to find bright spots and **bruits,** seen in subdural effusions and porencephalic cysts, respectively. (Bruits in non-anemic older children suggest increased ICP or an intracranial intravenous shunt or aneurysm.)

During early and late childhood the examination of the head follows the same procedures as that for adult patients (see Chapter 3):

Eyes. Sometimes it is difficult to examine the eyes of the newborn because the orbicularis muscle tends to contract in response to any attempt to open them. The best technique for inspecting the eyes of a newborn is to hold the baby upright in your extended arms, fixing the head in the midline. This position gives you a good view of the newborn's eyes because it forces the eyes to open. Turn the baby to the one side and then the other, and you will note that the eyes move in the direction in which you are turning. When rotation stops, the eyes will look in the opposite direction, followed by a few nystagmoid movements. During the first 10 days of life, the eyes do not move but remain fixed ("doll's eye" test). Inspect the iris for coloboma and the sclera for subconjunctival hemorrhages and the blink reflex to light (present at birth). Observe the inner epicanthal folds. **Funduscopic examination** must be delayed until the 2- or 6-month visit. **Test the optical blink reflex** to light by shining a bright light in the eyes.

During early childhood it is very important to try to determinate the presence of **amblyopia,** reduced vision in one normal eye caused by disuse. It is caused by a disconjugate fixation (strabismus) or by an eye refractive error of 1.5 diopters or more (anisometropia). To evaluate, you need to perform the **Hirschberg test.** This test consists of attracting the patient's attention to a light held at the level of your head and pointing it toward the child's eyes. As the child's eyes are fixed on the light, note the light's reflection on each cornea, and, with your other hand holding the child's head, turn the light to the left and then to the right while maintaining the child's head in a fixed position. Look for a corneal reflection. This must be symmetrically placed—note any asymmetry observed on the light's reflection. The reflection can detect, for example, left **isotropy** (inward eye deviation) or left exotropia (**outward deviation**). Children in late childhood are evaluated in the same way as adult patients.

Ears. During infancy it is very important to inspect the form and position of the auricles. Deformed or low-set auricles are related to congenital defects, especially renal agenesis or anomalies. **Test the hearing** by inspecting the infant's reaction (blinking eyes) to a sudden sharp sound such as snapping fingers, clapping hands, or a ringing bell. The acoustic blink reflex can be elicited during the first 2 or 3 days of life. It may disappear momentarily and after the stimulus has been performed a few times so that the infant becomes accustomed to it. Usual responses are as follows: at 2 weeks of age, the infant may jump; at 10 weeks, he or she may respond by momentary cessation of body movements; and at the age of 3–4 months the eyes and head will turn toward the source of the sound. During early childhood the examination becomes a little more difficult due to less cooperation from the patient. The exploration of ear canals with otoscopy is almost the same as that for adult patients (see Chapter 3).

Nose and throat. Remember that newborns are nasal breathers. Be careful when you examine them. Use your own approach to examining the child. Examining the baby when he or she is crying gives a good opportunity to observe the pharynx. You must make a quick inspection of the throat. Don't forget the sequence of tooth eruption: at 7 months, most infants have two upper and lower incisors; four more are added every 4 months. At the age of 15 months the infant has 12 teeth and, by 23 months, a full complement of 20. **Transilluminate** the frontal sinuses by placing a light above them in a dark room. If the sinuses are normal, you should see a faint glow of light transmitted through the bone outlining the frontal sinus on the same side. Transillumination is absent or diminished when sinusitis is present. In general, the examination techniques are the same as those for adult patients (see Chapter 3).

Review the following examples:

HEENT *(Extended format)*

Head: Normocephalic and free of visible lesions. Anterior and posterior fontanelles are soft—normal—tender. Sagittal suture palpable, mildly depressed. Chvostek's sign present.
Eyes: Conjunctivae clear without abnormalities. Prominent inner epicanthal folds, optical reflex to light present and normal.
Ear, nose and throat: Pinnae appear low-set. Ear canals showed no evidence of scarring or deformity on inspection. Nasal septum showed no deviation. Tongue was midline and appeared prominent.

HEENT

Conjunctivae clear without abnormalities or signs of infection.
Funduscopic exam: without signs of exudates or arteriolar venous nicking.
Ear canal, tympanic membranes normal.
Oropharynx moderate, injected retropharyngeal mucosa, without exudate.

HEENT

Head normal. Eyes reveal bilateral redness + injected conjunctivae + for mild exudate. ENT normal.

Neck

Notes on the neck follow the same general order and approach as adult written medical notes. Concentrate on problems related to the thyroid gland. Hypothyroidism is more common during infancy and childhood; hyperthyroidism and thyroiditis are more common during adolescence and preadolescence. For more information, see Chapter 3. Review the following examples:

Neck

Supple without bruit, thyroid gland normal.

Neck

Thyroid nodule 2 X 2 cm noted on the R side, painless with regular borders and non-mobile. Cervical nodes negative, no bruits detected.

Neck

Normal on inspection. Irregular L mass noted on palpation. Pain (−).

Chest

In general the physical examination of the chest, including the lungs and heart, is the same as that for adult patients. Some differences apply, such as the shape of the thorax of the newborn and young child, which normally is rounded and thin. The apical impulse, or point of maximal impulse (PMI), often is visible at the level of the 4th interspace until the age of 7 years, at which time it starts to be visible at the 5th intercostal space instead. On percussion, the heart appears larger because the heart is in a horizontal position. Sinus arrhythmia and premature ventricular contractions are quite common. Fifty percent of children develop an innocent murmur at some time during childhood. The **innocent murmur** is characterized as "innocent" because it appears during systole, lasts for only a short time, and is grade 3 or less in intensity. It is loudest along the sternal border, either in the 2nd or 3rd intercostal spaces or in the 4th or 5th intercostal spaces medial to the apex. Other organic murmurs (**non-innocent**) are caused by congenital or acquired heart disease, such as **rheumatic fever.**

It is important to familiarize yourself with normal values, according to age, in children (Table 7–4). Blood pressure measurement in children and infants is frequently omitted. Many clinicians erroneously judge it difficult to obtain blood pressure from an active child. However, when the procedure is properly explained, most children older than 3 years of age like the sphygmomanometer. For CSA exam purposes, the BP will be posed on the doorway information sheet.

Remember that the current ECFMG policy states that no children will be presenting as SPs. Considering this, you will not be able to perform a child's breast exam. As a reference, the breasts of both male and female newborns are often enlarged and engorged with secretion ("witch's milk") due to the maternal estrogen effect, which can last for 1 to 2 weeks. Breast development in girls normally occurs around age 11. Thelarche is the first phenotypic sign of puberty and occurs in response to the circulating estrogen. You need to teach the parent, caretaker, or the girl if this is the case, how to perform a breast and axillae self-examination. Determination of breast stage development (Tanner stages) is part of the physical (chest) examination. Problems, such as erythema, tenderness, dimpling, asymmetric masses or size, and axillary adenopathy, should be noted by the examiner, girl, or caretaker.

See the following examples for pediatric notes:

Chest: There is no evidence of superficial scars. A pectus excavatum was noted, no abnormal respiratory movements were noted.

Respiratory: Normal BS without any added sounds were noted.

Cardiac: Regular rate and rhythm. Normal S1 and S2, no murmur or gallop.

TABLE 7–4. Normal Values in Children

Age	Heart Rate	Systolic Blood Pressure*
Birth	140	50
6 mos	130	70
6–12 mos	115	90
1–2 y	110	95
2–6 y	103	100
6–10 y	95	110
10–14 y	85	115
16 y	85	120

Diastolic pressure reaches 60 mm Hg by 1 year and gradually increases during childhood to approximately 75 mm Hg.

*Approximate values taken from boys.

Chest

> **Resp:** There is tachypnea and obvious use of accessory muscles. Expiratory wheezing (+), crackles (−), dullness was noted.
> **Cardiac:** Tachycardia was noted with normal S1 and S2. Murmurs(−).

Chest

> **Respiratory:** There is tachypnea with ↓ respiratory movements on the R. side. Dullness with ↓ BS was noted on the middle area of the R. lung.
> **Cardiac:** Tachycardia was noted (+) regular pulse, normal S1 and S1. Murmurs (−).

Abdomen

The physical examination of the abdomen uses the same maneuvers as for adult patients, but with some variations on normal anatomy depending on the age of the patient. As discussed earlier, the approach to children varies depending on their age and health status. Children are almost universally ticklish; talking or distracting them before proceeding to any maneuver is very helpful. The main differences among infants, children, and adults are as follows.

During **infancy,** the abdomen is protuberant. The edge of the liver, the tip of the spleen, both kidneys, and the bladder are palpable. The descending colon is easily felt and may present as a sausage-like mass in the left lower quadrant. See Table 3–20 for the differences among adults and children with renal masses. Be aware of some common problems that affect infants. Infants are prone to umbilical hernias, ventral hernias, and recti diastasis.

During the **childhood** years, the liver and spleen are easily palpated in most children. The edge of the liver normally is felt 1 cm to 2 cm below the right costal margin, and the spleen also is easily palpable, with sharp edges. The examination of inguinal hernia in this age group is similar to that for adult patients.

See the following examples of medical notes:

Abdomen

> NL bowel sounds, soft, non-tender, without hepatosplenomegaly and masses.

ABD

> There is an ↑ in bowel sounds. Tenderness and pain were noted on superficial palpation of the LRQ. (+) rebound and guarding was noted.

ABD

> NL abdominal bowel sounds. Medial regular abdominal mass of 6 × 10 cm was palpated. (−) pain or tenderness was noted.

Genitalia

Per the ECFMG®, you are not allowed to perform a genital or rectal examination during the CSA exam. The following are some examples of medical notes for genital exams, **but they are for reference only:**

Genitourinary

> Normal penis on inspection; there are no testicles palpated on the scrotum. An inguinal mass was palpated on the L. side.

GU

(+) urethral discharge. Two inguinal lymph nodes palpated bilaterally. Testes were normal.

Genital

Tanner III scale pubic hair development. A small testicular mass/cyst was palpated on the R.

Neurologic Examination

The neurologic examination of an infant differs greatly from that of an adult. It is not the purpose of this book to review the clinical exam at this age in great detail, but we will mention some important aspects. First, the neurological assessment of infants relies on history (**developmental skills**) and inspection. Second, the central nervous system at birth is not well developed and works at subcortical levels. Cortical functions develop slowly after birth and cannot be tested completely until early childhood.

There are several specific reflex activities, known as **infantile automatism,** that are found in the normal newborn and disappear gradually over the course of the first months. Inspection is a very important tool used by the clinician to determine whether or not any problem is present. Noting the general appearance, positioning, activity, and alertness of the infant gives a general idea of the neurologic status. You can discuss these patterns with the parent or caretaker. Review the following parameters:

Motor function: Observe the infant's general movements. Note the muscle tone or any abnormality such as flaccidity or spasticity.

Sensory exam: Note the movements (withdrawn?) or facial expression as you touch and stimulate extremities or other parts of the body.

Cranial nerves (CNs): Test as for adults, but some difficulties will be obvious when you examine CNs I, II, VIII, and IX–XII (due to poor cooperation of the infant).

Reflexes: The spinal reflex responses, such as deep tendon reflex (DTRs) and plantar responses, are variable because development of the corticospinal pathway is still incomplete. Some reflexes are present at birth and are fully developed, such as the Babinski response and abdominal and anal reflexes:

1. **Plantar Babinski.** This reflex can be elicited by stimulating the lateral aspect of the sole from the heel to the ball of the foot, curving medially across the ball using a sharp object, such as a key (see Chapter 3). The Babinski response is abnormal in children older than 2 years of age, but may be found in normal children before this age.
2. **Abdominal reflex.** Stimulate the abdominal region using a sharp object or wisp of cotton (to test light touch). Observe a fine abdominal muscle contraction.
3. **Anal reflex.** Stimulate the perianal region with a sharp object, such as a tooth stick. Observe anal sphincter contraction. (You are never allowed to perform this test during the CSA exam.)

Infantile automatisms are present at birth or appear shortly thereafter. They have a prognostic value for the integrity of the CNS. The automatisms include the following:

1. **Blinking reflex,** in which the eyelids close to light. This normally disappears after the first year.
2. **Acoustic blink reflex,** in which both eyes blink to sharp loud noise. The time of disappearance is variable.
3. **Palmar grasp reflex.** Place your index fingers and press against the child's palmar surfaces. A positive response consists in one flexion of all of the child's fingers grasping your finger. Compare both hands. This reflex normally disappears at 3 or 4 months of age. Persistence of this reflex beyond 4 months may suggest cerebral dysfunction.

4. **Rooting reflex.** With your forefinger, stimulate the perioral skin of the corner of the child's mouth. Normal response consists of the infant opening his mouth and turning his head to the stimulated side. This reflex disappears at 3 or 4 months. Absence of this reflex indicates severe generalized or CNS disease.

5. **Trunk incurvation.** Stimulate one side of the baby's back along a paravertebral muscle. A normal response is a curving of the trunk toward the stimulated side. This normally disappears at 2 months.

6. **Placing response.** Hold the baby upright from behind by placing your hands under the baby's arms. The normal response is of alternate stepping in response to dorsal contact of one foot with the table. The timing of disappearance of this response is variable. Abnormalities may indicate spastic paraplegia.

7. **Tonic neck reflex.** Turn the baby's head to one side, holding the jaw over his shoulder. The normal response consists of an extension of the arm and leg on the side to which the head is turned, and flexion of the opposite leg and arm. This reflex may be present at birth, but usually disappears at 6 months. It is considered abnormal when the reflex is elicited each time it is evoked.

8. **Moro response.** This stimulus is elicited by any stimulus that suddenly moves the head in relation to the spine. It is normal at birth, but persistence of this reflex beyond 4 months may indicate neurologic disease. Asymmetric response in the upper extremity may suggest hemiparesis, brachial plexus injury, or clavicle fracture.

The neurologic examination during the childhood years is quite similar to that for adult patients (see Chapter 5), but some adaptations must be made for pediatric patients. For example stereognosis, vibration, position, two-point discrimination are not useful or completely developed in patients younger than 5 years old.

See the following examples of pediatric neurologic notes:

Neurologic

Alert, well oriented × 3. Cranial nerves normal. Motor 5/5. Sensory intact to pin, vibration, and proprioception. Deep tendon reflexes were 3/4. Plantar reflexes downgoing.

Neuro

Alert, well oriented × 3. CNs NL. Motor 5/5. Sensory intact to pin, vibration, and proprioception. DTR 3/4. Plantar reflexes ↓.

Neuro

Normal Moro's, blinking and palmar grasp reflexes. Motor and sensory function normal. No flaccidity was noted.

Neuro

There is normal movement on extremities except on the L. upper limb. There is pain on palpation on the L. clavicle. Other infantile responses were normal.

DIFFERENTIAL DIAGNOSIS

Limit yourself to five differential diagnoses. See the examples in Chapter 3.

DIAGNOSTIC WORKUP

Limit to enumeration of five differential diagnoses. See the examples in Chapter 3.

8

CSA Summary Review

This chapter reviews the most important CSA formats and provides examples of written notes that you will have to do on the CSA exam. As a final footnote, remember to stay calm and try to be well organized. At this point in your preparation for the CSA exam, you should be less anxious than before.

The cases that you will see on the day of the CSA exam are common scenarios. They are not likely to be complicated or unusual like the ones on the USMLE boards; let the biochemistry and pathophysiology rest in the back of your brain for a while. We encourage you to memorize the formats for written notes used in this book and accommodate them to the cases presented to you on the CSA exam. Remember that any section of a format may be individualized to suit each patient or your own notes. Use your own criteria, case by case.

Use the abbreviations that you are most familiar with. You can refer to the Appendix of Abbreviations at the back of this book, and you can also go to the ECFMG® website (www.ecfmg.org) to see some of the abbreviations they recommend. If you are accustomed to any particular diagram, only use it if it is going to save you time during the composition of your notes. Before entering the examination room, be mentally prepared to perform and complete the following objectives:

1. Focus on the chief complaint (CC), age, and any abnormalities in vital signs; this information is on the doorway information sheet. If you consider any of this information pertinent, write it on the blank paper provided for you.
2. Knock on the door before entering the examination room. Then introduce yourself to the standardized patient (SP).
3. Give the SP an opportunity to explain freely to you the CC. Make eye contact with the SP when you talk to him or her.
4. Make the appropriate notes you consider pertinent during the interview on the blank sheet of paper provided.
5. Before examining the patient, wash your hands or put on gloves.
6. Perform the clinical exam. Be polite and courteous in any maneuvering. Do not repeat painful maneuvers. Assist the patient/SP in any change of position during the examination.
7. Explain the findings and probable diagnosis to the patient. Do not use complicated medical terminology.
8. If you are considering ordering any laboratory studies, tell the SP why.
9. Answer any questions the patient has.
10. End your session when you consider it pertinent. Do not extend your maneuvering and questioning. Remember that you can finish your session before the entire 15 minutes is up and use any extra time to compose the written medical note!

You can elaborate in many ways on your written note. Try to be well organized in your questioning and maneuvering, and on the written note. Some patients may require a detailed, focused examination; others require only a general exam. Regardless, it is very important always to try to be concise in dialogue and questions. For example, if you have a patient who states that he is suffering from impotence, you need to look for problems that could be related to that, such as hypertension or diabetes. Detailed questioning regarding medications is very important, especially if you think that his problem may be related to that (e.g., sexual dysfunction due to clonidine treatment). In this case a detailed medical history regarding medications is very important and the physical exam is only complementary.

During the CSA exam, after you finish the encounter with your SP, you will compose a patient note. Blank forms to compose your medical note will be in a tray close to your desk outside the examining room. The format of a CSA blank patient note—as well as a completed patient note—can be found on the ECFMG website (www.ecfmg.org).

In the rest of this chapter, we summarize the written note formats and provide some examples of the kinds of cases you will encounter on the CSA exam. Review the following formats and written notes.

GENERAL MEDICAL EXAM: FORMAT AND CSA NOTES

A) MEDICAL HISTORY
1. Chief complaint (CC)
2. History of the present illness (HPI)
3. Past medical history (PMH)
4. Social history (SH)
5. Family history (FH)
6. Review of systems (ROS)

B) PHYSICAL EXAMINATION
1. General examination (GE)
2. HEENT
3. Neck
4. Chest ---► *Respiratory system*
       ---► *Heart*
5. Abdomen
6. Male genitalia
7. Neurologic
8. Musculoskeletal
9. Other

C) DIFFERENTIAL DIAGNOSIS
–Plans for dif. diagnosis (1-5)

D) DIAGNOSTIC WORKUP
–Plans for diagnosis (1-5)
–Plans for rectal/pelvic/female breast

FIGURE 8–1. Format for a medicine, family practice, or surgery note. Some information about the CC will be provided for you on the doorway information sheet as an opening scenario. You may or may not include it on your written medical note. For CSA purposes, you are not allowed to perform a genital, rectal, or female breast exam. HEENT = head, eyes, ears, nose, throat.

CASE 1

17-year-old male patient with headache.
Vital signs: P: 85/min, T: 37°C (98.5°F), R: 12 resp, BP: 125/80.

Medical History
CC: Mike is a 17 yo w. male patient stating he has a frontal headache.
HPI: He reports that he was well until 3 days ago when he started having an intermittent frontal bilateral headache that radiates to the occipital region. He describes it as not localized to any side, not pulsatile, and not related to an aura. He states that he is worried about the next football session because he is the chief team coordinator.
FH: Both parents are healthy. Grandfather died of stroke.
PMH: He describes himself as healthy. Immunizations are up to date. No recent trauma event was reported.
SH: He lives in a middle class neighborhood. He does not smoke, denies use of EtOH and other drugs.
ROS: Unremarkable.

Physical Examination
Gen: Patient appeared well. Vital signs: HR: 85/min, T:37°C, R: 12 resp/min, BP: 125/80.
HEENT: Conjunctivae normal, pupillary reflexes were normal. ENT were NL.
Neck: Palpation of the paravertebral neck muscles exacerbated the localized pain and tenderness that radiates to the occipital region bilaterally.
Chest: Normal BS, no wheezing, no crackles. Normal heart sounds, normal rhythm, normal S1, S2.
Abdomen: Normal on inspection, soft without tenderness.
Neuro: Alert, well oriented × 3. CNs normal. Motor 5/5. Sensory intact to pin, vibration, and proprioception. DTRs were 3/4. Plantar reflexes ↓.

Differential Diagnosis
1. Tension headache
2. Migraine headache
3. Headache secondary to sinus infection

Diagnostic Workup Plan
1. CBC
2. Electrolytes
3. Head x-rays; Cadwell, Watters
4. ESR

CASE 2

22 year old black male with sore throat and chills.
Vital signs: P: 82/min, T: 38.5°C (101.3°F), R: 14 resp, BP: 120/80.

Medical History

CC: Samuel is a 22 yo b. ♂ patient stating he has a sore throat and chills.

HPI: He states that he was well until a week ago when he started to have a mild sore throat. 4 days ago it was accompanied with chills and fever, mild abdominal pain. Denies diarrhea and cough. He also noted mild changes in skin coloration and other vague symptoms like anorexia, asthenia, and adynamia.

FH: Both parents alive, apparently healthy.

PMH: Tonsillectomy at 7 yo. He denies the use of medications, EtOH, and illicit drugs. Smoking (+), 2–3 cig./weekends.

SH: He is a pre-med college student. He states that recently has been visiting the city's children's hospital. He states having a friend with the same symptoms.

ROS: Cardiovascular—Unremarkable

Respiratory—Sore throat, no cough

GI—Abdominal fullness sensation. No diarrhea, no pain.

Immune system—Refers cervical tenderness. No opportunistic infections.

Physical Examination

Gen: P: 82/min., T: 38.5°C, R: 14 resp, BP: 128/80.

HEENT: Pupillary reflexes were NL. Mild jaundice was noted on conjunctivae. Throat shows an erythematous pharynx, tonsils not visible, no purulent exudates.

Neck: Cervical nodes are palpable, tender, and painful bilaterally.

Chest: Normal BS, no wheezing, no crackles. Normal heart sounds, normal rhythm.

Abdomen: Normal on inspection. Bowel sounds are present. Mild tenderness on palpation on the RUQ, hepatomegaly of 5 cm was detected on palpation and percussion.

Skin: Mild jaundice was noted.

Neuro: Unremarkable.

Differential Diagnosis

1. Mononucleosis
2. Hepatitis
3. Gilbert syndrome
4. Sickle cell disease
5. Post-hepatic causes of jaundice

Diagnostic Workup Plan

1. CBC
2. Peripheral blood smear
3. LFT: AST, ALT, alk. phosp, GGT, Bilirubin D/T, PT, PPT
4. Cell solubility test

CASE 3

70 year old forgetful female.
Vital signs: P: 85/min, T: 37°C (98.6°F), R: 12 resp, BP: 140/90 mm Hg.

Medical History

CC: Norma is a 70 yo ♀ stating that she is all right!

HPI: Pt is brought by her daughter because of forgetfulness during the past two years. Pt states that she is OK although her daughter disagrees with her. There weren't any particular precipitant events, such as CVA events or recent falls. Patient's daughter states that she confuses people's names and on one occasion she walked outside her home and took a bus to an undetermined direction. She was found by the police department.

FH: (+) for stroke, CAD, and dementia.

PMH: HTN dx 20 years ago, tx with propanolol bid. Hip fx two years ago. Cholecystectomy 15 years ago.

SH: EtOH during weekends up to 40–50 yo. No smoking. Lives with her daughter and grandsons. She was a housewife, her husband died 18 years ago.

ROS: Cardiovascular—SOB and dyspnea tx with digoxin 0.125 mg, M–F. + Bilateral edema on legs. Functional classification class II.

Physical Examination

Gen: VS: P: 85/min, T: 37°C, R: 12/min, BP: 140/90.

HEENT: Head and pupillary reflexes were NL, ↓ hearing bilaterally, ENT normal.

Neck: Supple, no masses, no bruises, no JVD.

Chest: No crackles, no wheezing, no abnormal BS. Heart sounds were rhythmic, S3 sound was heard on LSB, PMI impulse was palpated.

Abdomen: R subcostal scar was noted on inspection. NL bowel sounds, no masses, no ascites or visceromegaly.

Neuro: MMSE 20/30, CNS grossly within normal limits. Motor: Muscle tone was normal, strength was 5/5 to all muscles tested.

Sensory: Normal to pin and vibration. DTR 2/4.

Differential Diagnosis

1. Alzheimer's disease
2. Dementia
3. Multi-infarct dementia
4. Hypothyroidism
5. Vitamin B12 deficiency

Diagnostic Workup Plan

1. CBC
2. Electrolytes + BUN
3. Vitamin B12/folic acid levels
4. TSH, T4
5. Head CT scan

OBSTETRICS AND GYNECOLOGY: FORMAT AND CSA NOTES

A) OBSTETRIC/GYNECOLOGIC HISTORY
1. Chief complaint (CC)
2. History of the present illness (HPI)
3. Present pregnancy (PP)
4. Obstetric and gynecologic history (Ob/GynH)
5. Past medical history (PMH)
6. Social history (SH)
7. Family history (FH)

B) PHYSICAL EXAMINATION
1. General Examination (GE)
2. HEENT
3. Neck
4. Chest ···► *Breasts*
    ···► *Respiratory system*
    ···► *Heart*
5. Abdomen
6. Gynecologic and obstetric examination
7. Extremities ···► check edema
8. Neuro ···► check hyperreflexia

C) DIFFERENTIAL DIAGNOSIS
−Plans for dif. diagnosis (1-5)

D) DIAGNOSTIC WORKUP
−Plans for diagnosis (1-5)
−Plans for rectal/pelvic/female breast

FIGURE 8–2. Format for an obstetrics and gynecology note. You can disregard the present pregnancy section if the patient is presenting with only a gynecologic problem. Also, indicate a breast and gynecologic exam on the Diagnostic Workup Plan, but for CSA purposes do not perform these exams. HEENT = head, eyes, ears, nose, throat.

CASE 1

> 22 year old female having abdominal pain.
> **Vital signs:** P: 100 beats/min, T: 37.8°C (100.4°F), R: 12 resp/min, BP: 125/85.

Medical History

Chief C.: Lisa is a 22 yo w. female patient having abdominal pain.

HPI: She was fine until last night when she perceived a progressive midabdominal colic type pain. The pain was initially vague and then ↑ in intensity and moved progressively to LLQ. She refers to missed menses since 3 weeks ago. There is no urinary disturbance.

PMH: UTIs on two occasions. Denies STD.

Social: She is a college student and lives alone with roommate. She works part-time in a fast food restaurant close to her college.

OB & GYN Hx.: Menarche at 12 yo. LMP: 12/13/99, Pap smear never done. Birth control with condoms with single partner, bloody spot 10 days ago.

FH: Both parents alive, they are healthy.

ROS: Unremarkable.

Physical Examination

Gen: P: 100/min, T: 37.8°C, R: 15 resp, BP: 110/70. Appeared age stated.

HEENT: Pupillary reflexes were NL. ENT were NL

Neck: Unremarkable.

Chest: Normal breath sounds, no wheezing, no crackles. Normal heart sounds, normal rhythm, normal S1, S2.

Abdomen: Bowel sounds are present but ↓ in frequency. Pain and tenderness on superficial palpation on LLQ. + rebound and guarding signs.

Skin: Somewhat pale.

Differential Diagnosis

1. Ectopic pregnancy
2. Adnexal torsion
3. Bleeding of corpus luteum
4. PID

Diagnostic Workup Plan

1. Pelvic/speculum examination
2. Quantitative serum hGC
3. Pelvic ultrasound
4. CBC
5. Laparoscopy

CASE 2

37 year old pregnant patient who came for prenatal care.
Vital signs: P: 89 beats, T: 37°C (98.6°F), R: 14 resp, BP: 140/90.

Medical History
Chief C: No complaints, although reports sporadic headaches.

HPI: Maria is 35 yo hispanic ♀ who is in her second trimester of pregnancy. She missed her prenatal visits for two months due to foreign travel. She mentions not having any major complaints, although she has had sporadic frontal headaches since 3 weeks ago.

Present pregnancy: Mild low back pain, normal appetite and sleep. No mood alterations, pregnancy was planned. LMP was 12/13/99; EDC: 9/20/00; GA: 22 weeks; G: 6 P 2-2-1-4

PMH: UTIs on two occasions. Denies STD.

Social: Married with two children. Works as social worker for the city of Houston.

OB & GYN Hx: Last abortion was 2 years ago. Menarche at 11 yo, Pap smear yearly, last results normal. Sexual activity since 18 yo. No contraception.

FH: Both parents alive, they are healthy.

ROS: Unremarkable.

Physical Examination
Gen: P: 80 beats, T: 37.8°C, R: 15 resp, BP: 140/90.

HEENT: Pupillary reflexes were normal, normal funduscopy. ENT NL.

Neck: NL on inspection and palpation.

Chest: Normal BS bilaterally. Normal heart sounds, normal rhythm, normal S1, S2.

Abdomen: Uterine size 20 cm; FHR 110/min.

Normal bowel sounds, no hepatosplenomegaly detected on palpation. Leopold's revealed a longitudinal lie position with apparent occiput presentation.

Neuro.: Well oriented X 3, normal speech, CNs, motor and sensory exam unremarkable. Patellar reflexes (4+/5).

Skin: NL

Differential Diagnosis
1. Pre-eclampsia
2. Gestational HTN
3. Chronic HTN
4. HELLP syndrome

Diagnostic Workup Plan
1. Urinalysis: 24-hr urinary prot and volume
2. BUN/Cr
3. LFTs: ALT, AST, total bilirubin
4. CBC + peripheral blood smear

NERVOUS SYSTEM: FORMAT AND CSA NOTES

A) COMPLETE NEUROLOGIC EXAMINATION
1. Mental status examination and speech
2. Cranial nerves examination
3. Motor system examination:
   tone, strength, coordination
4. Sensory system examination
5. Reflexes examination

B) MENINGEAL TESTS
1. Kernig test
2. Brudzinski test

FIGURE 8–3. The format of a neurologic exam.

CASE 1

28 year old female patient with tingling hand.
Vital signs: P: 75/min, T: 37°C (98.6°F), R: 15 resp, BP: 130/85.

Medical History

CC: Mrs. Stevenson is a 28 yo ♀ patient having R. tingling hand.

HPI: She was well until a year ago when she started having sporadic tingling over her 1st, 2nd and 3rd digits. She was relatively well until last night when she started having the same sensation, but this time there wasn't any relief after the usual rest. She reports that tingling is worse over the index and middle finger. This sensation worsens at work when she types on the computer keyboard. No radiation or pain was described.

PMH: NIDDM (−), HTN (−), arthritis (−). Meds: oral contraceptives.

FH: Unremarkable.

SH: She works as a computer programmer at a technical institute.

ROS: Cardiovascular, GI, renal, and endocrine unremarkable.

Physical Examination

Gen: P: 70/min, T: 36.5°C, R: 15 resp, BP: 110/80

HEENT: Conjunctivae were normal, pupillary reflexes were NL. ENT were NL.

Neck: Normal on inspection, palpation and auscultation.

Chest: Heart: NL rhythm, NL heart sounds. BS were NL without added sounds.

Abdomen: Soft without tenderness or pain on palpation.

Neuro: CNs normal. Strength was 5/5 bilaterally on upper limbs. Sensory was intact to pin, vibration, and proprioception. Brachioradialis reflex was 2/4 bilaterally. Other unremarkable.

Musc: No pain or tenderness on flexion and extension movements of the R. hand at the wrist. No abnormalities on lateral movements. Phalen's and Tinel's signs were (+) on the R. hand.

Differential Diagnosis

1. Carpal tunnel syndrome
2. Ulnar radiculopathy
3. Cervical radiculopathy

Diagnostic Workup Plan

1. CBC
2. Electrolytes
3. ESR
4. Electromyography

CASE 2

| 67 year old female patient complaining of diminished strength. |
| **Vital signs:** P: 100/min, T: 37°C (98.6°F), R: 16 resp/min, BP: 140/90 |

Medical History

Chief C: Margaret is a 67 yo b. ♀ stating that she has ↓ strength in her L. side.

HPI: She was well until last night while she was bathing when she had a sudden loss of conscious. She doesn't remember more about the incident until she awoke on a paramedic bed. Initially she wasn't able to talk but she regained her speech when she arrived at the hospital. At the present time she refers having ↓ strength and paresis on her L. side.

FH: (+) for stroke, HTN, and NIDDM.

PMH: HTN dx 15 years ago; tx Enalapril 10 mg QD. Denies falls or head trauma. NIDDM was dx 10 years ago; tx NPH insulin 30 U/day. Hysterectomy at 45 yo due to myomatosis.

SH: She consumes 5 oz of wine a day. Smokes 2 pkg/day. Other drugs (−).

ROS: Cardiovascular—No palpitations, no dyspnea, angina no MI hx. Respiratory—No CHF, dyspnea. Renal/genital—Nephropathy due to urolithiasis.

Physical Examination

Gen: P: 100 beats/min, T:37°C, R: 16 resp, BP: 140/90

HEENT: Conjunctivae and pupillary reflexes were normal. Mild L. facial deviation.

Neck: A grade 3 carotid bruit on the L. side.

Chest: Respiration—NL BS, no wheezing, no crackles. Cardiac—NL heart sounds, NL S1, S2. No murmurs, NL rhythm.

Abdomen: NL on inspection, soft without tenderness.

Neuro: Alert, well oriented×3. CN: mild L deviation of lip commissurae. Motor: 5/5 on R. side and intact to pin, vibration, and proprioception. On the L. side strength 3/5 on upper and lower limbs. ↓ sensation to pin on the L. side. Reflexes:

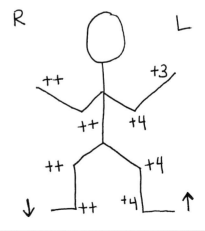

Differential Diagnosis
1. TIA
2. RIND
3. Stroke
4. Cerebral hemorrhage

Diagnostic Workup Plan
1. CT scan of head
2. Carotid Doppler ultrasound
3. ECG
4. Echocardiogram

PSYCHIATRIC EXAM: FORMAT AND CSA NOTES

A) PSYCHIATRIC HISTORY
1. Chief complaint (CC)
2. History of the present illness (HPI)
3. Psychiatric history
4. Past medical history (PMH)
5. Social history (SH)
6. Family history (FH)
7. Developmental psychiatric history
8. Review of systems (ROS)

B) MENTAL STATUS EXAMINATION (MSE)
1. General aspects
2. Mood and affect (emotions)
3. Speech
4. Perception
5. Thought
6. Cognitive and intellectual functions (Mini-Mental Status Examination [MMSE])
7. Impulse control
8. Judgment and insight

C) DIFFERENTIAL DIAGNOSIS
–Plans for dif. diagnosis (1-5)

D) DIAGNOSTIC WORKUP
–Plans for diagnosis (1-5)

FIGURE 8–4. The format of a psychiatric history and mental status examination (MSE).

CASE 1

23 year old male hearing voices.
Vital signs: P: 90/min, T: 37°C (98.5°F), R: 15/min, BP: 130/85.

Medical History

CC: Joe is 23 yo w. ♂ who says he is hearing voices.

HPI: This young man is admitted due to first-time appearance of hallucinatory voices. The patient was well until 2 months ago when he started having delusions of reference by friends and neighbors. His personality has progressively been changing during this period of time, until 2 days ago when he started hearing voices.

FH: Both parents died three months ago in an MVA. They were apparently healthy.

Psych Hx: There was no hx of previous psychiatric problems.

PMH: Tonsillectomy at 12 yo, clavicle fracture at 8 yo.

SH: EtOH (−), smoking and drug abuse (−). He worked as a librarian at the county public library.

Developmental: He states that his early childhood was a happy one. He describes his mom as a domineering and imposing person, his father was very friendly although without character. He does not have a girlfriend.

Mental Status Examination

Gen: P: 90/min, T: 37°C, R: 15 resp/min, BP: 130/85. Appearance poorly groomed. Eye contact inappropriate. Attitude was cooperative.

Mood: Euthymic.

Affect: Flat.

Speech: NL in rate, tone and volume. Rhythm changes spontaneously. No echolalia or word salad.

Perception: Hallucinatory voices are presently described by the patient as "orders that are trying to control him." There weren't any illusions.

T/P: LOA (+), FOI (+), Tangential (+).

T/C: Feeling of unreality (+), delusion of reference (+). No suicidal ideation.

Cognitive: Alert, well oriented, poor concentration and abstract thinking. Intelligence appears average.

Judgment and insight: Fair.

Differential Diagnosis

1. Schizophreniform disorder
2. Brief psychotic disorder
3. Schizoaffective disorder
4. Schizophrenia
5. Intoxication

Diagnostic Workup Plan

1. CT head scan
2. VMA
3. CBC
4. Electrolytes
5. Urinary toxicologic studies

CASE 2

> 48 year old female with insomnia.
> **Vital signs:** P: 70/min, T: 37°C (98.5°F), R: 14 resp/min, BP: 130/80.

Medical History

CC: Melissa is a 48 yo female stating having insomnia since a year ago.

HPI: She was well until a year ago, when her husband died suddenly. She has difficulty sleeping, she constantly dreams and remembers him. She mentions loss of appetite, weakness, and weight loss.

FH: Mother alive with RA. Father died 20 years ago.

Psych Hx: No hx of depression, compulsions, or schizophreniform syndromes.

PMH: Laparotomy at 40 yo due to ovarian cyst. Current medication include midazolam 1 mg QD.

SH: Smoking (−), drinks socially although reports that she has recently been drinking at night trying to induce sleep. She lives alone, she has one daughter who recently moved to Boston for college. She works as a supervisor at a grocery store.

Developmental: She states having good recollections about her childhood and adolescence. She describes herself as a dependent person. She married her high school sweetheart at 18.

Mental Status Examination

Gen: P: 70 beats/min, T: 37°C, R: 14 resp/min, BP: 130/80.

Appearance: Appeared age stated, relatively well groomed, looks tired.

Activity: Cooperative, activity ↓.

Attitude: Appropriate.

Mood: Euthymic.

Affect: Sad.

Speech: NL in rate, tone, rhythm, and volume.

Perception: No illusions, no hallucinations.

T/P: Logical and goal directed, LOA (−), FOI (−), Tangential (−), Neologisms (−).

T/C: Sadness, no suicidal ideation, no delusions.

Cognitive: MMSE 30/30.

Impulse control: Normal.

Judgment and insight: Normal.

Differential Diagnosis

1. Normal grief
2. Depression
3. Bipolar disorder
4. Schizoaffective disorder

Diagnostic Workup Plan

1. CBC
2. Electrolytes
3. Dexamethasone suppression test

PEDIATRICS: FORMAT AND CSA NOTES

A) PEDIATRIC MEDICAL HISTORY
 1. Chief complaint (CC)
 2. History of the present illness (HPI)
 3. Past medical history (PMH)
    ···► *Birth history*
        + Prenatal, natal, and neonatal history
    ···► *Feeding history*
    ···► *Growth and development*
    ···► *Immunizations and*
        screening procedures
    ···► *Childhood illnesses*
    ···► *Social development*
 4. Social history (SH)
 5. Family history (FH)
 6. Review of systems (ROS)

B) PHYSICAL EXAMINATION
 1. General examination (GE)
 2. HEENT
 3. Neck
 4. Chest ···► *Respiratory system*
       ···► *Heart*
 5. Abdomen
 6. Genital/inguinal examination
 7. Neurologic
 8. Musculoskeletal

C) DIFFERENTIAL DIAGNOSIS
 –Plans for dif. diagnosis (1-5)

D) DIAGNOSTIC WORKUP
 –Plans for diagnosis (1-5)
 –Plans for rectal/pelvic/female
 breast

FIGURE 8–5. The format for a pediatric note.

CASE 1

1 year 6-month old child with mild fever and rash.

Vital signs: P: 100/min, T: 38°C (100°F), R: 15 resp/min.

Medical History

CC: Chris is an 18 month old infant with fever, malaise, anorexia and rash.

HPI: Patient's mother states that he was well until a day ago when he started having irritability, anorexia, and general malaise. She gave him Children's Tylenol to control fever, but this morning she noted the appearance of pruritic rash on his trunk.

FH: Father died 9 months ago in Kosovo war. Mother apparently healthy. His paternal grandfather died of stroke.

PMH: Normal at birth, maternal feeding for 6 months, immunizations are up to date. Chris's mother states that he had been screened for lead and anemia 6 months ago. He feeds himself using a spoon; he can stack 3 blocks and put small objects into a bottle.

Medications—Children's Tylenol (acetaminophen) TID.

SH: His father was a Marine. He has one sister who is 4 years old.

ROS: Mother reports that the patient has only sporadic common colds; denies asthma, bronchiolitis, pneumonia, GI infections or previous hospitalizations.

Physical Examination

Gen: P: 100/min, T: 37.5°C, R: 15 resp/min.

HEENT: Conjunctivae were moderately hyperemic, pupillary reflexes were normal. ENT were OK.

Neck: Examination of the neck was unremarkable.

Chest: Characteristic papules and scabs were noted over the trunk. Clear BS, no wheezing, and no crackles. Heart sounds were normal rhythm, no murmur.

Abdomen: On inspection, vesicles with scabs were noted. Normal auscultation and palpation. No hepatosplenomegaly was noted.

Skin: Papules and vesicles were noted over the trunk and began to spread peripherally over the arms and legs. Rash lesions are characterized by having papules, some vesicles look cloudy and form scabs.

Differential Diagnosis

1. Chickenpox (varicella)
2. Rubella
3. Roseola infantum

Diagnostic Workup Plan

1. CBC
2. ESR
3. Tzanck test

CASE 2

8 year old child who came for a well child visit
Vital signs. P: 90/min, T: 37°C (98.6°F), R: 16 resp/min

Medical History

CC: Carlos is an 8 yo hispanic child who came with his mother for a well child visit.

HPI: Patient's mother states that they just moved to town because her husband started his postgraduate studies at the local university. She reports that Carlos is a healthy kid and he has no major complaints at this time. He came for a well child visit.

FH: His grandfather is diabetic, alive; grandmother with HTN.

PMH: Normal at birth, breastfeeding for 6 months, weaning at 5. Immunizations are up to date, but HBV (−). She was asked about lead screening and she doesn't know. She was also asked about PPD. She reports that Carlos was vaccinated with BCG at birth but she doesn't know about PPD test. Carlos speaks little English, although he is learning very fast.

SH: He comes from a well-educated family. At the present time he lives at the university housing village, he has one younger sister.

ROS: Unremarkable.

Physical Examination

Gen: Well appearance, healthy boy. P: 90/min, T: 37°C, R: 16 resp/min.

HEENT: Conjunctivae, pupillary reflexes, ENT were normal.

Neck: Normal on inspection, palpation and auscultation.

Chest: There is an obvious pectus excavatum noted on inspection. Inspiratory movements were NL. BS were NL, no crackles, no wheezes. PMI was noted on the 5th intercostal space and anterior axillary line. NL S1 and S2 were noted.

Abdomen: Normal bowel sounds, no pain or tenderness, no hepatosplenomegaly.

Musk: Normal muscle mass, NL strength.

Differential Diagnosis

1. Normal school age child
2. Pectus excavatum

Diagnostic Workup Plan

1. CBC
2. Blood lead
3. PPD

9

Residency Programs: The Next Step

APPLICATION PROCESS

This chapter presents information that may be helpful when you apply for a residency position. Although once you have passed the exams (i.e., USMLE Steps 1 and 2, TOEFL, and the CSA exam), you are in a good position for entering residency, the greatest challenge is still to come. After you have passed one or two USMLE exams, you can begin your search for a residency program. The initial process is confusing, and there is no single source that provides all the necessary information, especially in regard to several changes that have been made to the process of certification and application since 1997.

You probably have heard of **matching, applications,** and **interviews,** but no single, official source about the process is available. Most of what you learn comes from other, more experienced IMGs. Most of the process works well for U.S. graduates, but it can be more challenging in certain ways for IMGs. As you will find in almost any country, nationals may receive preferences that a foreigner does not. Therefore, IMG applicants are urged to apply for a greater number of positions than U.S. graduates in hopes of obtaining an interview. (U.S. graduates, on average, apply to 20 programs and obtain, on average, 10 to 15 invitations to interview. An IMG may apply to 80 or more programs.) Furthermore, your need to learn about residency programs is more acute than that of U.S. graduates. Some U.S. graduates have spent time during their electives in other institutions and already know that they want to apply to them when they finish their studies; obviously, they can get a good letter of recommendation, and then they have preference. Until 1996, the process of applying for residency had stayed basically the same, and followed these five major steps:

1. Contact available residency programs directly, as posted in the "**green book**" (the *Graduate Educational Directory*) and **FREIDA** (*Fellowship and Residency Electronic Interactive Database;* **www.ama-assn.org/cgi-bin/freida/freida.cgi**). The green book is an annually updated catalog published by the American Medical Association (AMA) that lists all training programs recognized by the Accreditation Council for Graduate Medical Education (ACGME). It is not as complete as FREIDA, which is an annually updated PC-based database of residency programs produced by the AMA.
2. Get applications and requirements from residency program directors.
3. Mail applications and other paperwork as required by each residency program.
4. Obtain and complete an interview.

5. Participate in the National Residency Matching Program (NRMP), commonly known as **matching.**

Since 1997, there have been changes in the application process for some specialties. The first change is the implementation of the **Electronic Residency Application System (ERAS),** a universal way to contact program directors.

Until 1999, after enrolling and paying the fee, you received a software kit (diskettes) to install on a computer. Then you filled out the universal application format and chose the specialties from the ACGME program that you were interested in. Then you returned one of the diskettes to ECFMG® with your information and your letters of recommendation, transcripts, photo, and so forth to be scanned and sent via the Internet to the programs that you have selected. In the year 2000, the Association of American Medical Colleges introduced a web-based service—MyERAS—that transmits residency applications, letters of recommendation, Dean's letters, medical school transcripts, and so forth, from you and your school (for U.S. graduates) or from you and the ECFMG® (for IMGs) to the residency program directors who are using the Internet. After enrolling and paying the fee, you are given a "token" (a special code) so that you can access and register with MyERAS on-line. For information on this program, go to the following web site: **www.myeras.aamc.org.**

Most of the specialties participate in ERAS and no longer accept paper applications, although exceptions may be made by individual programs. It is important to remember that some individual hospitals do not participate in ERAS. According to the ERAS 2001 Application Manual, the specialties that participate in ERAS are:

Anesthesiology
Dermatology
Diagnostic radiology
Emergency medicine
Emergency medicine/internal medicine
Family practice
Internal medicine (preliminary and categorical)
Internal medicine/family practice
Internal medicine/pediatrics
Internal medicine/psychiatry
Obstetrics and gynecology
Orthopaedic surgery
Pathology
Pediatrics
Pediatrics/emergency medicine
Pediatrics/physical medicine and rehabilitation
Physical medicine and rehabilitation)
Psychiatry
Psychiatry/family practice
Surgery (preliminary and categorical)
Transitional year
Army and Navy PGY-1 positions

Note that internal medicine and surgery both list the terms **preliminary** and **categorical.** Preliminary programs provide 1 or 2 years of prerequisites for entry into advanced programs that require 1 or more years of clinical training. Categorical programs expect applicants who enter in their first postgraduate year to continue until they have completed training requirements for specialty certification, provided their performance is satisfactory (normally 3 to 4 years). The **transitional year** is a graduate year of training or flexible internship during which you can do rotations in different fields, such as obstetrics and gynecology, pediatrics, orthopaedics, anesthesiology, traditional medicine, and surgery.

The overall application process currently consists of the following steps:

1. Get the ERAS token so you can access MyERAS on the World Wide Web from the ECFMG®.
2. Contact each residency program for requirements, deadlines, and other important information.
3. Obtain and have an interview.
4. Participate in the National Residency Matching Program (NRMP).

The overall process of applying to residency programs has been streamlined. At the same time, it is more expensive and you are indirectly forced to apply to fewer programs than you would have done before. Through ERAS, the more programs you apply for in one specialty, the more expensive it becomes. The first 20 programs that you apply to cost a set amount of money; applying for 21 to 30 programs costs you twice as much (see current ERAS information on the web site at **www.aamc.org/eras**). ECFMG® makes it more difficult to apply to a wide variety of programs, which was easy to do with paper applications. If you have plenty of money you can still apply to all the programs, but this is not the case for most IMGs.

You are likely to have a better chance of obtaining a residency if you apply for several different specialties rather than applying to just one specialty.

We encourage you to contact the residency program directors before randomly choosing a hospital listed in MyERAS. You can contact the different program directors by writing directly to them or by sending an e-mail message. Using e-mail is cheap and fast, and it can give you a rough idea of the programs for which you may be a tentative candidate.

Some programs have special regulations for IMGs. For example, they may specify minimum passing scores and may want to know how many times you have taken the USMLE board exams, any previous experience in U.S. hospitals, research experience, etc. Some simply do not accept IMGs, and some programs accept only U.S. citizens and green card holders. This information is important to know, so that you do not waste time and money applying to programs for which you are not even eligible. If you obtain this information in the MyERAS database before choosing your **hospital options,** it focuses your application on programs in which you have potential as a candidate. This will save you money and increase your chances of getting an interview.

We recommend that you start as soon as possible. July is a good time to start gathering information about the program requirements for IMGs, and by October you should have an idea of which programs will give you the best opportunity as an applicant.

Not all graduate programs post e-mail addresses in the green book or FREIDA. It is also possible to contact program directors by regular mail.

There is no particular predetermined background that is needed to be accepted in a residency program. Obviously, it is always helpful to have good scores on the USMLE boards, good grades in medical school, and good letters of recommendation.

IMMIGRATION

Visas

As an IMG residing in your home country, you most likely are not familiar with the paperwork that you will need to deal with when you find a residency position in the United States. The purpose of this section is not to explain the process for obtaining different visas, but to try to give you a broad overview of what is available. If you are a U.S. citizen or permanent resident you can skip this section. However, if you earned your medical degree outside the U.S., for medical licensing purposes, you are considered an IMG and it does not matter if you are a U.S. citizen or a permanent resident.

The following types of visas permit a foreign graduate medical trainee to study in the U.S.

Exchange Visitor (J-1). This is the most common visa obtained by IMGs who are starting graduate medical education in the U.S. The visa is good for the length of time typically required to complete the program, and is limited to a maximum of 7 years. It is not possible to change from this status to another, even if you marry an American citizen. The only way to work in the U.S. after finishing your graduate medical education is through a process known as the **waiver.** This means that the Immigration and Naturalization Service (INS), the U.S. agency that deals with immigration issues, will exonerate the applicant from his commitment to return to his home country after finishing his residency in a U.S. hospital. This process is complicated, and it recently has become harder to obtain a waiver.

Temporary Worker (H-1B). To be a candidate for this visa you need to pass the USMLE Step 3. Under this visa status you can legally work in the U.S. for the institution that is sponsoring you. You may travel outside of the U.S., and there are no restrictions against obtaining permanent residency (green card) in the U.S. (This is a separate process called Labor Certification; it does not interfere with your H1-B visa status.)

Student Optional Practice Training (F-1). Students with F1 status may be authorized for up to 12 months of practical training after completion of studies for an appointment that can be completed in 12 months. This can be appropriate for a foreigner who has already studied medicine in the U.S. and received a U.S. medical degree.

Persons of Extraordinary Ability (O-1). This category is for individuals with extraordinary ability demonstrated by sustained national or international acclaim. These people come into or remain in a graduate medical program to apply their research clinically or to enhance or improve their techniques by acquiring related skills. You can get a green card through this process, but you must be prepared to prove your "extraordinary ability" by providing evidence such as proof of publication in major medical journals, awards, and accomplishments.

Before you decide which visa to apply for, you must define your goals. **What do you want to do after finishing the residency?** If you do not have plans to work in the U.S. and you intend to return to your home country, the J-1 visa status is fine. If, however, you wish to work in the U.S. after finishing your residency, the J-1 visa can be a problem. If you have plans to stay in the U.S. after finishing your graduate medical training, it is preferable to enter the residency program under the H-1B visa, because under this visa there is no obligation to return to your home country. It can be renewed for up to 6 years. The only drawback is that you have to continue to work for the same employer who sponsored you to get the H-1B visa. In other words, if you want to change employers in the course of these years you will have to reapply again for a new H-1B visa.

It is important to know that not all hospital programs sponsor H-1B visas—some sponsor only J-1 visas, some sponsor both J-1 and H-1B visas, and others sponsor only J-1 but allow you to handle the paperwork for the H-1B visa. Remember that immigration issues are handled by the federal government and that any immigration attorney in any state can handle the visa paperwork.

Qualifying Exams

The following are important aspects that are not discussed in the ECFMG®/USMLE bulletin.

The USMLE exams are **licensing exams.** A foreign physician who has passed only the USMLE Steps 1 and 2, the Test of English as a Foreign Language (TOEFL), and the Clinical Skills Assessment exam and holds an ECFMG® certificate does not have a complete license to practice in the U.S., and, therefore, is not eligible to apply for an H-1B visa. To become a candidate for the H-1B visa you must pass the USMLE Step 3 as well. To enter into graduate medical education in the U.S., it is necessary to have an ECFMG® certificate (and to get this certification, you need to pass USMLE Steps 1 and 2, TOEFL, and CSA exam). The USMLE tests are a common evaluation route for all applicants who want to practice and be trained in the U.S. The USMLE Step 3 is administered by each state's licensing authorities, which may impose additional requirements for taking this exam in their jurisdictions. The USMLE Step 3 is *not* a prerequisite for applying to residency programs, and it does not affect your chances of being accepted. U.S. graduates usually enter the residency program just after passing the USMLE Step 2. They then take the USMLE Step 3 sometime during their residency, depending on the requirements of the state in which they are doing the residency and the state in which they plan to practice. You need to fulfill the requirements of the state in which you are eligible and/or which state you want to practice medicine.

Requirements of Individual States

Individual states do not all have the same rules for IMGs as for U.S. graduates. Some states, for example, do not allow you to take the USMLE Step 3 before you have not had at least 1 year of graduate medical education in the U.S. (In some states this policy holds true for both U.S. graduates and IMGs.) Other restrictions may include, for example, the number of times that you have taken USMLE Steps 1, 2, and 3; currently, there is no mention of a quota for the CSA exam. Some residents at institutions in a state that does not permit them to take the USMLE Step 3 arrange to take it in another state where they are eligible. After they finish their residency, they can endorse the USMLE Step 3 exam to the state that they are planning to be licensed in (Remember: Every state has it's own requirement).

There are approximately 10 states that allow IMGs to take the USMLE Step 3 before they have had graduate medical education in a U.S. or Canadian hospital; typically, states require 6 months to 2 years of residency education. We strongly recommend that you visit the following website—**www.fsmb.org**—to obtain current information from each individual licensing authority. Please note that requirements are subject to change without notice.

Finally, the USMLE Step 3 is not the last test that you will need to take. Other requirements depend on the jurisdiction in which you are planning to practice and may include other exams, such as oral examinations, American specialty board certification, and so forth.

ON-LINE RESOURCES

The challenges confronting IMGs trying to get into a U.S. residency program are increasing every day. No one really knows at this time what the impact of the CSA exam will be on the prospects of IMGs. (For example, in the near future, more program directors may start to have passing the CSA exam as a requirement, and this would affect those IMGs who were certified by the ECFMG® before July 1998.) It appears that in the future, program directors will ask for the current requirements stated by the ECFMG® at the time of selection. This policy will affect the IMGs who are currently certified by the ECFMG®. We will have to wait and see what changes will occur in the requirements.

Both official and unofficial information is available on the Internet. The following list offers some on-line sources that may be helpful:

Educational Commission for Foreign Medical Graduates
www.ecfmg.org
This is the official home page of the ECFMG®. On this web site you can find updated and current information about the USMLE and CSA exams and ERAS. It contains important information and links with other web pages related to the NRMP, residency programs, and certifications. You can order information booklets and application materials through this site.

National Resident Matching Program (NRMP)
http://nrmp.aamc.org/nrmp
This is the official web site that you must use if you are participating in the NRMP.

To log onto this web page, you need to be registered for the match and you need to use your NRMP code and PIN number. Several important dates are specified for **listing your rank order list, making changes on your post office or e-mail address,** seeing the **results of the match,** and seeing the **filled and unfilled positions.** The **"scramble"** takes place the day after the final match results are posted; candidates who did not match may find a position in the scramble. The filled and unfilled positions are posted on this site at a specific date and time. Applicants may contact hospitals directly, and contracts may be offered by telephone. For the appropriate dates, see the most recent NRMP bulletin.

Test of English as a Foreign Language (TOEFL)
www.toefl.org

This home page is very useful and efficient. You can find detailed information about the new Computer-Based TOEFL (CBT). You can reach the Educational Testing Service to ask questions concerning booklets and ways to order or download the TOEFL CD-ROM sampler.

American Medical Association (AMA)
www.ama-assn.org

The main page for the AMA contains updated information about new policies, accreditation, membership information, etc. It includes important links to FREIDA, ERAS, and NRMP. Go to the main page, click on "sitemap" on the top bar, and scroll down to Medical Education.

Fellowship and Residency Electronic Interactive Database (FREIDA)
http://www.ama-assn.org/cgi-bin/freida/freida.cgi

This is an important web page where you can search residency programs for the current year by region. It provides the same information as the green book. If you become an AMA member, you can obtain a mailing label address from the residency programs. This way you can make several copies of a form letter requesting hospital information. It saves you a great deal of time.

Electronic Residency Application System (ERAS)
www.aamc.org/about/progemph/eras

This web page offers detailed information about the specialties that are listed in ERAS and about the participating programs. When you use ERAS you can follow your application through the Applicant Document Tracking System. As an IMG, you first must contact the ECFMG® to obtain the ERAS Token and current information about ERAS.

Immigration and Naturalization Service (INS)
www.ins.usdoj.gov

This is the official web page of the INS. A broad explanation of the different visas can be found in this page. You can download useful INS forms, and if the form that you are looking for is not downloadable, you can order it on-line.

USMLE Forums
http://go.to/usmleforums

This forum is a place to discuss issues related to entering a residency program. You can discuss issues related to the Match, ERAS, externships, observerships, interviews, residency programs, and visa issues for IMGs. Get tips, share your experiences, and buy and sell books related to residency issues.

Pinoy IMG
www.pinoyimg.net

This is a useful web page with information about the USMLE boards, the TOEFL test, the CSA exam, residency, interviews, fellowships, and immigration issues. You will find other important information such as unfilled residency positions, forums discussion groups, useful links, and so forth.

Appendix of Abbreviations

COMMON ABBREVIATIONS USED IN UNITED STATES HOSPITALS

ABG = Arterial blood gases
Abd = Abdomen
ACE = Angiotensin-converting enzyme
aCL = Anticardiolipin (*antibody*)
ACT = Activated clotting time
ACTH = Adrenocorticotropic hormone
ADH = Antidiuretic hormone
ad lib = As desired, freely
adm = Admission
AF = Atrial fibrillation
AFB = Acid-fast bacilli
AIDS = Acquired immune deficiency syndrome
AKA = Above knee amputation
alb = Albumin
alk phos = Alkaline phosphatase
ALL = Acute lymphoblastic leukemia
ALS = Amyotrophic lateral sclerosis
AMI = Acute myocardial infarction
AML = Acute myelogenous leukemia
ANA = Antinuclear antibody
ANCA = Antineutrophil cytoplasm antibody
ANLL = Acute nonlymphocytic leukemia
Anti-SMA = Anti-smooth muscle antibody
A&P = Auscultation and percussion
AP = Anteroposterior
APS = Anti-phospholipid syndrome
APTT = Activated partial thromboplastin time
AR = Aortic regurgitation
ARC = AIDS-related complex
ARDS = Acute respiratory distress syndrome
ARF = Acute renal failure
asa = Aspirin
ASHD = Arteriosclerotic heart disease
ASLO = Anti-streptolysin O
ATG = Acute tubular necrosis

AVM = Arteriovenous malformation
B = black
BACOD = Bleomycin, doxorubicin (*Adriamycin*), cyclophosphamide, vincristine (*Oncovin*), dexamethasone
BACOP = Bleomycin, doxorubicin (*Adriamycin*), cyclophosphamide, vincristine (*Oncovin*), prednisone
BBB = Bundle branch block
BC = Blood culture
BCG = Bacillus Calmette-Guerin
BCP = Birth control pill
BE = Barium enema
bid = Two times a day
bilat = Bilateral
billi = Bilirubin
BKA = Below knee amputation
BM = Bowel movement
BMR = Basal metabolic rate
BP = Blood pressure
BPH = Benign prostatic hypertrophy
bpm = Beats per minute
BR = Bed rest
BRP = Bathroom privileges
BS or bs = Breath sounds
BSA = Body surface area
BSO = Bilateral salpingo-oophorectomy
BTL = Bilateral tubal ligation
BUN = Blood urea nitrogen
BW = Body weight
Bx = Biopsy
Ca = Cancer
Ca^{+2} = Calcium
CAB = Coronary artery bypass
CABG = Coronary artery bypass grafting
CAD = Coronary artery disease
CAF = Cyclophosphamide + doxorubicin (*Adriamycin*) + 5-fluoroulacil
CAT = Computed axial tomography

cath = Catheterization

CAV = Cyclophosphamide + doxorubicin (*Adriamycin*) + vincristine

CBC = Complete blood count

CBD = Common bile duct

cc = Cubic centimeter

CC = Chief compliant

CCr = Creatinine clearance

CCU = Cardiac care unit

CEA = Carcinoembryonic antigen

CHD = Coronary heart disease

CHF = Congestive heart failure

CHOP = Cyclophosphamide + doxorubicin (*Adriamycin*) + vincristine (*Oncovin*) + prednisone

CI = Cardiac index

CIE = Counterimmunoelectrophoresis

CK = Creatine kinase

CK-MB = Creatine kinase, myocardial band

CLL = Chronic lymphocytic leukemia

cm = Centimeter

CM = Costal margin

CMF = Cyclophosphamide + methotrexate + 5-fluorouracil

CML = Chronic myelogenous leukemia

CMV = Cytomegalovirus; controlled mechanical ventilation

CNS = Central nervous system

CO = Cardiac output

c/o = Complaining of

COPD = Chronic obstructive pulmonary disease

CPAP = Continuos positive airway pressure

CPK = Creatine phosphokinase

CPR – Cardiopulmonary resuscitation

Cr = Creatine

CRH = Corticotropin-releasing hormone

C/S = Culture and sensitivity

CSF = Cerebrospinal fluid

C/sec = Cesarean section

CT = Computed tomography

CTS = Carpal tunnel syndrome

Cu = Copper

CV = Cardiovascular

cva = Costovertebral angle

CVA = Cerebrovascular accident

CVP = Central venous pressure

CXR = Chest x-ray

DA = Developmental age

D&C = Dilation and curettage

D&S = Dilation and suction

DGI = Disseminated gonococcal infection

DHPG = Ganciclovir

DIC = Disseminated intravascular coagulation

DKA = Diabetic ketoacidosis

DM = Diabetes mellitus

DNA = Deoxyribonucleic acid

DPT = Diphtheria pertussis tetanus

DR = Delivery room

DTs = Delirium tremens

DU = Duodenal ulcer

DUB = Dysfunctional uterine bleeding

DVT = Deep venous thrombosis

D5W = Dextrose (5%) in water

Dx = Diagnosis

EBV = Epstein-Barr virus

ECF = Extracellular fluid

ECG = Electrocardiogram

ED = Emergency department

EDC = Estimated date of confinement

EDTA = Ethylene diamine tetraacetate

EEG = Electroencephalogram

EENT = Eyes, ears, nose and throat

EGD = Esophago-gastroduodenoscopy

EIA = Electroimmunoassay

EJV = External jugular vein

EKG = Electrocardiogram

ELISA = Enzyme linked immunoassay

EMG = Electromyogram

EMT = Emergency medical technician

ENT = Ears, nose, throat

EOM = Extraocular muscles

EPO = Erythropoietin

EPS = Extrapyramidal symptoms

ER = Emergency room

ERCP = Endoscopic retrograde cholangiopancreatography

ERS = Evacuation retained secundines

ESR = Erythrocyte sedimentation rate

ESRD = End-stage renal disease

ETOH = Alcohol

Ext = Extremities

f = female

FSB = Fasting blood sugar

FDP = Fibrin degradation product

Fe = Iron

FFP = Fresh frozen plasma

FH = Family history

FHR = Fetal heart rate

FNA = Fine-needle aspiration

FOI = Flight of ideas

FS = Frozen section

FSH = Follicle-stimulating hormone

FTA-ABS = Fluorescent treponemal antibody absorbed

FTI = Free thyroxine index

5-FU = 5-fluoracil

FUO = Fever of undetermined origin
fx = Fracture
g = Gram
GA = Gestational age
GB = Gallbladder
Gc = Gonococcus
GERD = Gastroesophageal reflux disease
GFR = Glomerular filtration rate
GGT = γ-glutamyltransferase
GGTP = γ-glutamyl transpeptidase
GI = Gastrointestinal
glu = Glucose
GN = Glomerulonephritis
G6PD = Glucose-6-phosphate dehydro-
    genase
GPA = Guided percutaneous aspiration
GSW = Gunshot wound
GTT = Glucose tolerance test
GU = Genitourinary
GVHD = Graft-versus-host disease
Gyn = Gynecology
H2 = Histamine-2
HAV = Hepatitis A virus
Hb = Hemoglobin
HBcAg = Hepatitis B core antigen
HBsAg = Hepatitis B surface antigen
HBIG = Hepatitis B immune globulin
HBP = High blood pressure
HBV = Hepatitis B virus
HCO3⁻ = Bicarbonate
Hct = Hematocrit
HCV = Hepatitis C virus
HDL = High-density lipoprotein
HDV = Hepatitis D virus
HEENT = Head, eyes, ears, nose, and
    throat
H/H = Hemoglobin/hematocrit
h-hCG = Human chorionic gonadotropin
HIV = Human immunodeficiency virus
H&L = Heart and lungs
HLA = Human leukocyte antigen
HMG-CoA = 3-hydroxy-3-methylglutaryl
    coenzyme A
HNP = Herniated nucleus pulposus
H2O = Water
H2O2 = Hydrogen peroxide
h/o = History of
H&P = History and physical exam
HPF = High power field
HPI = History of the present illness
hr = Hour
HR = Heart rate
HSV = Herpes simplex virus
ht = Height
HTN = Hypertension

Hx = History
I&D = Incision and drainage
IBD = Inflammatory bowel disease
IBS = Irritable bowel syndrome
ICP = Intracranial pressure
ICU = Intensive care unit
IDDM = Insulin dependent diabetes mel-
    litus
IFA = Immunofluorescent assay
Ig = Immunoglobulin
ILD = Interstitial lung disease
IM = Intramuscularly
inj = Injection
INR = International normalized ratio
IOP = Intraocular pressure
IQ = Intelligence quotient
IUD = Intrauterine device
IV = Intravenous
JVD = Jugular venous distention
JVP = Jugular vein pulse
k = kilogram
KJ = Knee jerk
KUB = Kidney, ureter, and bladder
l or L = Left
LA = Left atrium
LAD = Left axis deviation
LAHB = Left anterior hemiblock
lap = Laparotomy
lb = Pound
LBP = Low back pain
LBBB = Left bundle branch block
LDH = Lactate dehydrogenase
LDL = Low-density lipoprotein
LES = Lower esophageal sphincter
LFT = Liver function test
LGV = Lymphogranuloma venereum
LH = Luteinizing hormone
LHRH = Luteinizing hormone-releasing
    hormone
LLL = Left lower lobe
LLQ = Left lower quadrant
LMP = Last menstrual period
LNMP = Last normal menstrual period
LOA = Loose of associations
LP = Lumbar puncture
LPHB = Left posterior hemiblock
LSB = Left sternal border
LUL = Left upper lobe
LUQ = Left upper quadrant
LVH = Left ventricular hypertrophy
m = Murmur; male; meter
MAC = Mycobacterium avium complex
MAO = Monoamine oxidase
MAP = Mean arterial pressure
MBC = Minimum bactericidal concentra-

tion

MCA = Middle cerebral artery

MCL = Midclavicular line

MCP = Metacarpophalangeal

MCV = Mean corpuscular volume

MEN = Multiple endocrine neoplasia

MERSA = Methicillin-resistant *Staphylococcus aureus*

mg = Milligram

MI = Myocardial infarction

MIC = Minimal inhibitory concentration

min = Minute

MMSE = Mini-Mental Status Exam

mod = Moderate

MOPP = Mechlorethamine, vincristine (Oncovin), procarbazine, prednisone

MPGN = Membrane proliferative glomerulonephritis

MRI = Magnetic resonance imaging

MRSA = Methicillin-resistant *Staphylococcus aureus*

MVA = Motor vehicle accident

N = Normal

NA = Not applicable

NaHCO3 = Sodium bicarbonate

Neuro = Neurologic

NIDDM = Non-insulin-dependent diabetes mellitus

NG = Nasogastric

NGU = Nongonococcal urethritis

NH3 = Ammonia

NKA = No known allergies

NKDA = No known drug allergies

NL = Normal limits

NPH = Normal pressure hydrocephalus

NPH = Neutral protamine Hagedorn (*Insulin*)

NPO = Nothing by mouth

NS = Normal saline

NSR = Normal sinus rhythm

NSAID = Nonsteroidal antiinflammatory drug

NSR = Normal sinus rhythm

NTG = Nitroglycerin

OB = Obstetrics

OB&Gyn = Obstetrics and gynecology

op = Orally

ophth = Ophthalmology

OR = Operating room

ortho = Orthopedics

oz = Ounce

P = Pulse

P2 = Pulmonic second sound

PaCO2 = Partial pressure of CO2 in arterial blood

PaO2 = Partial pressure of O2 in arterial blood

P&A = Percussion and auscultation

PA = Posterior-anterior; pulmonary artery

pap = Papanicolaou

para = Number of pregnancies

PAWP = Pulmonary artery wedge pressure

PBC = Primary biliary cirrhosis

PCO2 = Carbon dioxide tension

PCP = *Pneumocystis carinii* pneumonia

PCR = Polymerase chain reaction

PCWP = Pulmonary capillary wedge pressure

PE = Physical exam

ped = pediatric

PERLA = Pupils equal and reactive to light and accommodation

PFT = Pulmonary function test

PGE = Prostaglandin E

PH = Past history

PI = Present illness

PID = Pelvic inflammatory disease

PIP = Proximal interphalangeal

PKU = Phenylketonuria

PMI = Point of maximal impulse

PMP = Previous menstrual period

PM&R = Physical medicine and rehabilitation

PMR = Polymyalgia rheumatica

PND = Paroxysmal nocturnal dyspnea

PO = By mouth

PO2 = Oxygen tension

PPD = Purified protein derivative

PROM = Premature rupture of membranes

PRL = Prolactin

prn = As needed

PSA = Prostate-specific antigen

PSC = Primary sclerosing cholangitis

PSGN = Post streptococcal glomerulonephritis

PSVT = Paroxysmal supraventricular tachycardia

Psych = Psychiatry

pt = Patient

PT = Prothrombin time

PTT = Partial prothrombin time

PTC = Percutaneous transhepatic cholangiography

PTCA = Percutaneous transluminal coronary angioplasty

Pth = Pathology

PTH = Parathormone

PTU = Propylthiouracil

PUD = Peptic ulcer disease
PVC = Premature ventricular contraction
Px = Physical examination
q = Every
qd = Every day
qh = Every hour
qid = Four times daily
r or R = Right
R = Respirations
RA = Rheumatoid arthritis; right atrium
RBBB = Right bundle branch block
RBC = Red blood cells
RDS = Respiratory distress syndrome
RDW = Red cell distribution width
R&E = Round and equal
REM = Rapid eye movement
RF = Rheumatoid factor
Rh = Rhesus blood factor
RIND = Reversible ischemic neurologic deficit
RLL = Right lower lobe
RLQ = Right lower quadrant
RML = Right middle lobe
ROM = Range of motion
ROS = Review of system
RPGN = Rapidly progressive glomerulonephritis
RPR = Rapid plasma reagin
rpt = Repeat
rt-PA = Recombinant tissue plasminogen activator
R/T = Related to
rT3 = Reverse triiodothyronine
RTA = Renal tubular acidosis
RUL = Right upper lobe
RUQ = Right upper quadrant
RVH = Renovascular hypertension; right ventricular hypertrophy
S_1 = First heart sound
S_2 = Second heart sound
S_3 = Third heart sound
S_4 = Fourth heart sound
SA = Sinoatrial
SAH = Subarachnoid hemorrhage
SBE = Subacute bacterial endocarditis
SC = Subcutaneus
SGA = Small for gestational age
SGOT = Serum glutamic oxalacetic transaminase (Aspartate aminotransferase = AST)
SH = Social history
SIADH = Syndrome of inappropriate secretion of antidiuretic hormone
SGPT = Serum glutamic pyruvate transaminase (Alanine aminotransferase = ALT)
SL = Sublingual
SLE = Systemic lupus erythematosus
SLR = Straight leg raising
SLRT = Straight leg raising test
SOB = Shortness of breath
SOC = State of consciousness
SQ = Subcutaneous
SRM = Spontaneous rupture of membranes
stat = Immediately
STD = Sexual transmitted disease
supp = Suppository
Surg = Surgery
susp = Suspension
SVR = Systemic vascular resistance
SVT = Supraventricular tachycardia
Sx = Symptoms
syr = Syrup
T = Temperature
T_3 = Triiodothyronine
T_4 = Thyroxine
T&A = Tonsillectomy and adenoidectomy
tab = Tablet
TAH = Total abdominal surgery
TB = Tuberculosis
TBG = Thyroxine-binding globulin
Tbsp = Tablespoon
T/C = Throat culture
temp = Temperature
TIA = Transient ischemic attack
TIBC = Total iron binding capacity
tid = Three times daily
TIPS = Transjugular intrahepatic portosystemic shunt
TLC = Total lung capacity
TM = Tympanic membrane
TMP-SMX = Trimethoprim/sulfamethoxazole
TNM = Tumor node metastases
TMG = Toxic multinodular goiter
top = Topical
tPA = Tissue plasminogen activator
TP = Total protein
TPI = *Treponema pallidum* immobilization
TPN = Total parental nutrition
TPR = Temperature, pulse, and respiration
T3RIA = Triiodothyronine level by radioimmunoassay
T3RU = T3 resin uptake
TRH = Thyrotropin-releasing hormone
TRIG = Triglycerides
TSAb = Thyroid-stimulating antibodies
TSH = Thyroid-stimulating hormone

tsp = Teaspoon
TT = Thrombin time
TUR = Transurethral resection
TURP = Transurethral resection of the prostate
TV = Tidal volume
TWAR = *Chlamydia psittaci*
Tx = Therapy
U/A = Urinalysis
UFH = Unfractionated heparin
UGI = Upper gastrointestinal
US = Ultrasound
URAC = Uric acid
URI = Upper respiratory infection
UTI = Urinary tract infection
UV = Ultraviolet
vag hyst = Vaginal hysterectomy
VD = Venereal disease
VDRL = Venereal disease research laboratories (test for syphilis)
VER = Visual evoked response

VF = Ventricular fibrillation
VIP = Vasoactive intestinal polypeptide
VLDL = Very-low-density lipoprotein
VMA = Vanillylmandelic acid
VPC = Ventricular premature contraction
VO = Verbal order
vs = Visit
VS = Vital signs
w = White
WBC = White blood cell count
w/c = Wheel chair
WD = Well developed
WF = White female
WN = Well nourished
WNL = Within normal limits
WPW = Wolff-Parkinson-White syndrome
wt = Weight
x = Times
yo = Years old
ZDV = Zidovudine
Z-E = Zollinger-Ellison syndrome

COMMONLY USED SYMBOLS

@ = At
++ = Moderate amount
+++ = Large amount
0 = Zero, none
♀ = *Female* (BG: Find out the compositor code for the male and female symbols.)
♂ = *Male*
↑ = Increased
↓ = Decreased

= Number
< = Less than
> = Greater than
μm = Micron
μg = Microgram
+ = Positive, prescence
− = Negative
∅ = Absence of
Δ = Changes
° = Degree

Bibliography

—————•

Alvarado AJC: *Manual de Obstetricia, Major National University of Saint Marcos.* Lima, Peru, Gavelan-Hnos, 1992.

American Psychiatric Association: *Diagnostic and Statistical Manual of Mental Disorders,* 4e. Washington, DC, American Psychiatric Association, 1994.

April EW: *NMS Anatomy,* 2e. New York, John Wiley & Sons, 1990.

Bardes CL: *Essential Skills in Clinical Medicine.* Philadelphia, FA Davis, 1996.

Bates B: *A Guide to Physical Examination,* 3e. Philadelphia, JB Lippincott, 1983.

Beck W, Jr: *NMS Obstetrics and Gynecology,* 2e. New York, John Wiley & Sons, 1989.

Bhushan V, Hansen J: *First Aid for the Boards: A Student-to-Student Guide to the USMLE Step 1,* 3e. Norwalk, CT, Appleton & Lange, 1993.

Callahan TL, Caughey A, Heffner L: *Blueprints in Obstetrics and Gynecology.* Malden, MA, Blackwell Science, 1998.

Delph MH, Manning RT: *Propedéutica de Major,* 9e (From English edition of Major's Physical Diagnosis, 9e, WB Saunders). Mexico DF, Interamericana, SA de CV, 1985.

DeMyer WE: *Technique of the Neurologic Examination,* 4e. New York, McGraw-Hill, Inc, 1994.

Dworkin P: *NMS Pediatrics,* 2e. Baltimore, Williams & Wilkins, 1991.

Educational Commission for Foreign Medical Graduates: *Candidate Orientation Manual.* Philadelphia, 2001.

Epstein O, Perkin GD, de Bono DP, Cookson J: *Pocket Guide to Clinical Examination,* 2e. London, Mosby Wolfe, 1997.

Ewald GA, McKenzie C: *Manual of Medical Therapeutics,* 28e. Boston, Little Brown, 1995.

Fadem B: *BRS Behavioral Science,* 2e. Philadelphia, Harwal Publishing, 1994.

Fenner F, White DO: *Virología Medica,* 2e (From English edition of Medical Virology, Academic Press, Inc). Mexico DF, La Prensa Medica Mexicana, SA, 1987.

Flores FFJ: *Medicina Forense.* University of Monterrey, Mexico DF, Harla-Melo, SA, 1991.

Go A, Curet-Salim MT, Fullerton N: *First Aid for the Boards: A Student-to-Student Guide to the USMLE Step 2.* Stamford, CT, Appleton & Lange, 1996.

Godos CG, Venegas LN: *Actualización en Pediatría, Peruvian Boards of Physicians.* Lima, Peru, Educación Medica Continua, Colegio Medico del Perú, 1991.

Gray H: *Gray's Anatomy.* New York, Bounty Books, 1987.

Harrison TR: *Harrison's Principles of Internal Medicine,* 14e (CD-ROM). New York, McGraw-Hill, 1998.

Heger JW, Niemann JT, Roth RF, Criley JM: *House Officer Series: Cardiology,* 4e. Baltimore, Williams & Wilkins, 1998.

Hoppenfield S: *Exploración Física de la Columna Vertebral y las Extremidades* (From English edition of Physical Examination of the Spine and Extremities, Appleton-Century-Crofts). Mexico DF, El Manual Moderno, SA de CV, 1979.

Jones HW, Jones GS: *Tratado de Ginecología de Novak,* 11e (From English edition of Novak's Textbook of Gynecology, 11e, Lippincott Williams & Wilkins). Mexico DF, Interamericana, SA de CV, 1988.

Karp S, Morris J, Soybel D: *Blueprints in Surgery.* Malden, MA, Blackwell Science, 1998.

Lawrence PF: *Essentials of Surgery,* 2e. Baltimore, Williams & Wilkins, 1992.

Leal RP: *Infecciones Quirúrgicas,* Park Clinical Hospital, Chihuahua, Mexico, 1993.

Levinson WE, Jawetz E: *Medical Microbiology and Immunology,* 3e. Norwalk, CT, Appleton & Lange, 1994.

Myers AR: *NMS Medicine,* 2e. Baltimore, Williams & Wilkins, 1993.

Overturf GD: Pediatric bacterial CNS infections. *Infections in Medicine,* 8(1):17–25;1992.

Phillips D: *Longman Preparation Course for the TOEFL Test,* 2e. White Planes, NY, Addison-Wesley Publishing Company, 1996.

Pitchard J, McDonald P, Gant N: *Williams Obstetricia,* 3e (From English edition of Williams-Obstetrics, 11e, Appleton-Century-Crofts). Mexico DF, Salvat Editores, SA, 1990.

Pryse-Phillips W, Murray TJ: *Neurología Clínica* (From English edition of Essentials of Neurology, 2e, Medical Examination Publishing Company). Mexico DF, El Manual Moderno, SA de CV, 1984.

Pyle M, Munoz ME: *Cliffs Test of English as a Foreign Language Preparation Guide,* 5e. Lincoln, NE, Cliffs Notes, 1995.

Richard JM: *A Manual for the Beginning Ophthalmology Resident,* 3e. Rochester, MN, Custom Printing, Inc, 1980.

Rosales TC, Celestinon A, Tejada RL, Yamamoto JW, Wantanabe JY, et al: *Gastroenterología para Médicos Generales, Peruvian Boards of Physicians.* Lima, Peru, Educación Medica Continua, Colegio Medico del Perú, 1984.

Scully J, Bechtold D, Bell J: *NMS Psychiatry,* 2e. New York, John Wiley & Sons, 1989.

Stobo JD: *The Principles and Practice of Medicine,* 23e. Stamford, CT, Appleton & Lange, 1996.

Tortora G, Anagnostakos N: *Principios de Anatomía y Fisiología,* 3e (From English edition of Principles of Anatomy and Physiology, 3e, Harper & Row). Mexico DF, Harla Harper & Row Latinoamericana, 1984.

Wiechers EG: *Oftalmología.* Mexico DF, Interamericana-McGraw-Hill, 1995.

Wilson WR, Nadol JB Jr: *Manual de Otorrinolaringología* (From English edition of Quick Reference to Ear, Nose and Throat Disorders, JB Lippincott). Mexico DF, LIMUSA, SA de CV, 1987.

Index

—————•